Compartmental Analysis

Compartmental Analysis

Medical Applications and Theoretical Background

Editors
Fumihiko Kajiya, Okayama, *Shinzo Kodama*, Osaka, and *Hiroshi Abe*, Osaka

Associate Editors
Michitoshi Inoue, Mitsuyasu Kagiyama, Hiroshi Kita, Hideo Kusuoka, Hajime Maeda

77 figures and 13 tables, 1984

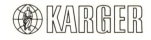

S. Karger · Basel · München · Paris · London · New York · Tokyo · Sydney

National Library of Medicine, Cataloging in Publication
Compartmental analysis, medical applications and theoretical background/editors, Fumihiko Kajiya, Shinzo Kodama, and Hiroshi Abe. —Basel; New York: Karger, 1984.
 1. Body Fluids-metabolism 2. Health Physics 3. Hemodynamics 4. Kinetics 5. Models, Biological 6. Systems Theory I. Abe, Hirosi, 1922- II. Kajiya, Fumihiko III. Kodama, Shinzo
 ISBN 3-8055-3696-8
 QH 324.8 C737

All rights reserved.
 No part of this publication may be translated into other languages, reproduced or utilized in any form or by any means, electronic or mechanical, including photocopying, recording, microcopying, or by any information storage and retrieval system, without permission in writing from the publisher.

© Copyright 1984 by Corona Publishing Co., Ltd., 4-46-10 Sengoku, Bunkyo-ku, Tokyo (Japan)
 Printed in Japan
 S. Karger AG, P.O. Box, CH-4009 Basel (Switzerland) has the exclusive distribution rights for all countries with the exception of Japan.

Contents

Preface VII
Introductory Remarks—Outline of Compartmental Analysis 1

Part 1
1 Estimation of Parameters in Compartmental Analysis
 . . . . (F. Kajiya, M. Kagiyama, N. Hoki and K. Kuwagoe) 9
2 Optimum Sampling for the Identificaton of Compartmental Systems
 . . . . (F. Kajiya, M. Kagiyama, M. Hori, K. Tsujioka and G. Tomonaga) 23
3 Structural Identifiability of Linear Compartmental Systems
 . . . . (H. Kusuoka, H. Maeda and S. Kodama) 36
4 Realization Problems in Linear Compartmental Systems
 . . . . (H. Maeda and S. Kodama) 47

Part 2
5 Radiocardiography . . . . . (A. Hirakawa, K. Minato and M. Kuwahara) 59
6 Hydrogen Gas Clearance Method for Regional Myocardial Blood Flow
 . . . . (M. Kinoshita) 66
7 Turnover of Serum Enzymes and its Application to Quantitative Assessment of Myocardial Infarct Size . . . . (M. Inoue, M. Hori and H. Abe) 79
8 Intrarenal Hemo- and Urodynamics Examined by Functional Images with I-131 Hippuran Renoscintigraphy . . . . . (T. Nishimura and K. Kimuma) 90
9 An On-line Monitoring System of Cerebral Blood Flow and Cerebral Oxygen Consumption . . . . (Y. Kuriyama) 97
10 The Time Course for the Decline in Miniature End-Plate Potential Frequency Following Tetanic Stimulation of the Motor Nerve
 . . . . (H. Kita, K. Narita and W. Van der Kloot) 106
11 Compartmental Analysis in Pulmonary Physiology, with Special Reference to the Distribution Function . . . . (T. Okubo) 119
12 Application of Kinetic Approaches to Water and Electrolyte (M. Nagasaka) 135
13 Application of Compartmental Model of Spleen Hemodynamics to in vivo Evaluation of Red Cell Rheology and its Destruction
 . . . . (Y. Takahashi and C. Uyama) 141
14 Multi-Compartmental System with Stochastic Input —Mathematical Formulation by the Ito Calculus and its Application to Health Physics—
 . . . . (S. Tatsunami, N. Yago and N. Fukuda) 156

Contents

15 Optimal Drug Administration Based on a Compartmental System
. . . (*H. Kusuoka, H. Maeda, S. Kedama, M. Inoue, H. Abe and F. Kajiya*) 166
16 Estimation of Transition Probabilities in Ischemic Heart Disease by Markov Model
(*M. Kagiyama, N. Hoki, G. Tomonaga, H. Kusuoka, Y. Ogaskwara and F. Kajiya*) 175
Index 187

Preface

Compartmental analysis is used to evaluate systems by outlining them with tracers, assuming that the system consists of compartments and the flow of tracer material depends on its concentration in the donor compartments. The objectives of compartmental analysis are to (a) conceptualize the system, (b) simplify complicated data, (c) predict the future behavior of the system under study, and (d) control the system optimally.

Compartmental analysis offers a useful mathematical model in the fields of medicine, basic as well as clinical, pharmacy, social science, behaviormetrics, ecology and econometrics. This book emphasizes the medical application of the compartmental model.

Though the compartmental model includes non-linear and variable coefficient forms, this book deals primarily with the linear, constant coefficient model, because the absorbing interest in compartmental models lies in its mathematical simplicity.

This book is divided into three parts: Introductory remarks outline compartmental analysis, i. e., define and characterize the system, review the historical perspective of compartmental analysis, the fields in which it is applicable, and the related system theoretical problems. In Part I, some important problems of the system theory encountered in compartmental analysis are discussed, since the system theory offers a mathematical background for the identification, evaluation and control of the compartmental system. Part II describes present and future applications of compartmental analysis to various medical fields. The applications include evaluations of blood flows in the heart, brain and spleen; of the process of intercellular communication of the lung and kidney functions; of body fluid and electrolyte metabolism, health physics, pharmacology, and the epidemiology of ischemic heart diseases. We believe that this book is useful and feasible not only in the medical but in other fields as well, since

Preface VIII

the basic idea and methodology are common to many fields.

Most of the contributors are members of scientific research projects (No. 00337049, 00555162, and No. 00537017) supported by the Ministry of Education, Science and Culture of Japan. The editors are highly indebted to all of the authors. Special thanks are due to Miss Yasuko Nishina for typing the manuscripts. The editors are also very grateful to the editorial staff of S. Karger AG and Corona Publishing Company, Ltd. In addition, one of the editors, Hiroshi Abe, is Secretary General of the 21st General Assembly of the Japan Medical Congress held in Osaka in 1983 and it is a special pleasure to see the book published at this commemorative occasion. We do hope that the book will contribute to the progress of health sciences.

Fumihiko Kajiya
Shinzo Kodama
Hiroshi Abe

Contributors

Hiroshi Abe, M. D., Ph. D., Department of Medichne, Osaka University Medical School, Osaka 553

Nobuo Fukuda, M. D., Ph. D., Division of Clinical Research, National Institute of Radiological Sciences, Chiba 280

Akina Hirakawa, M. D., Ph. D., Department of Biomedical Information, Kyoto University Hospital, Kyoto 606

Noritake Hoki, M. D., Ph. D., Department of Medical Engineering and Systems Cardiology, Kawasaki Medical School, Kurashiki, Okayama 701-01

Michitoshi Inoue, M. D., Ph. D., Department of Medicine, Osaka University Medical School, Osaka 553

Mitsuyasu Kagiyama, B. S., Computer Center, Kawasaki Medical School, Kurashiki, Okayama 701-01

Fumihiko Kajiya, M. D., Ph. D., Department of Medical Engineering and Systems Cardiology, Kawasaki Medical School, Kurashiki, Okayama 701-01

Kyoji Kawagoe, M. Eng., Application System Research Laboratory, Central Research Laboratories, Nippon Electric Co. Ltd., Kawasaki, Kanagawa 213

Kazufumi Kimura, M. D., Ph.D., Division of Nuclear Medicine, Osaka University Medical School, Osaka 553

Masahiko Kinoshita, M. D., Ph. D., Department of Medicine, Shiga Medical School, Otsu, Shiga 520-21

Hiroshi Kita, Ph. D., Department of Physiology, Kawasaki Medical School, Kurashiki, Okayama 701-01

Shinzo Kodama, Ph. D., Department of Electronics Engineering, Faculty of Engineering, Osaka University, Suita, Osaka 565

Yoshihiro Kuriyama, M. D., Ph. D., The Stroke Care Unit, National Cardiovascular Center, Suita, Osaka 565

Hideo Kusuoka, M. D., Department of Medicine, Osaka University Medical School, Osaka 553

Michiyoshi Kuwahara, Ph. D., Automation Research Laboratory, Kyoto University, Uji, Kyoto 611

Hajime Maeda, Ph. D., Department of Electronics Engineering, Faculty of Engineering, Osaka University, Suita, Osaka 565

Kotaro Minato, Ph. D., Department of Biomedical Information, Kyoto University Hospital, Kyoto 606

Masahito Nagasaka, M. D., Ph. D., Department of Medicine, Faculty of Medicine, Univer-

Contributors

sity of Tokyo, Tokyo 113

Kazuhiko Narita, M. S., Department of Physiology, Kawasaki Medical School, Kurashiki, Okayama 701-01

Tsunehiko Nishimura, M. D., Ph. D., Department of Radiology, National Cardiovascular Center, Suita, Osaka 565

Yasuo Ogasawara, M. Eng., Department of Medical Engineering and Systems Cardiology, Kawasaki Medical School, Kurashiki, Okayama 701-01

Takao Ōkubo, M. D., Ph D., Department of Medicine, Yokohama City University School of Medicine, Yokohama 232

Yutaka Takahashi, M. D., Ph. D., Division of Hematology, Tenri Hospital, Tenri, Nara 632

Shinobu Tatsunami, B. S., Radioisotope Research Institute, St. Marianna University School of Medicine, Kawasaki, Kanagawa 213

Go Tomonaga, M. D., Ph. D., Department of Medical Engineering and Systems Cardiology, Kawasaki, Medical School, Kurashiki, Okayama 701-01

Katsuhiko Tsujioka, M. D., Department of Medical Engineering and Systems Cardiology, Kawasaki Medical School, Kurashiki, Okayama 701-01

Chikao Uyama, Ph. D., Department of Electric Engineering, Faculty of Engineering, Kyoto 611

William Van der Kloot, Ph. D., Department of Physiology and Biophysics, School of Medicine, Health Sciences Center, State University of New York at Stony Brook, N. Y. 11794

Nagasumi Yago, Ph. D., Radioisotope Research Institute, St. Marianna University School of Medicine, Kawasaki, Kanagawa 213

INTRODUCTORY REMARKS
—— OUTLINE OF COMPARTMENTAL ANALYSIS ——

Fumihiko Kajiya, Shinzo Kodama and Hiroshi Abe

1. COMPARTMENTAL ANALYSIS

Basically, compartmental analysis is used to evaluate a system by measuring the input and output of a tracer introduced into that system. This method can be used to assess systems assumed to consist of one to several compartments and has a large number of applications not only in medicine and biology[1,2], but also in pharmacy, social science, behaviormetrics, econometrics and ecology[3]. This chapter outlines the characteristics, fields of application, and theoretical problems of the compartmental system[4].

2. COMPARTMENTAL SYSTEM

2.1 DEFINITION AND CHARACTERISTICS

Continuing interest in compartmental analysis is due to its mathematical simplicity. The system to be evaluated is divided into a number of compartments and the transport of substances from one compartment to another is described as a flux. The meaning of compartment, however, may differ, depending on the specific system being analyzed. For example, in some physiological systems, the compartment may correspond to a distribution pool of the tracer, such as a plasma or interstitial tissue fluid pool. At times, the term compartment is conceptual, and does not, therefore, have a real counterpart. For example, in a compartmental model the plasma pool does not completely coincide with its physiological definition.

The assumptions required for compartmental analysis are that the

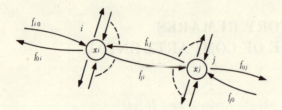

Fig. 1. Compartmental system: x_i is the amount of tracer in compartment i; f_{i0} the flow rate of tracer from the environment to compartment i; f_{0i} the flow rate from compartment i to the environment, and f_{ij} the flow rate from compartment j to compartment i.

tracer be distributed immediately and uniformly throughout a compartment and that the law of conservation holds true for the amount of tracer put into the system.

Letting the amount or concentration of tracer in compartment i be a state variable $\{x_i\}$, the dynamic equation of the tracer is represented by:

$$\frac{d}{dt}x_i = f_{i0} + \sum_{j \neq i} f_{ij} - \left(\sum_{j \neq i} f_{ji} + f_{0i}\right) \qquad (1)$$
$$x_i(0) = x_i^0, \quad i = 1, 2, \cdots, n,$$

where x_i^0 is the initial value of x_i; f_{i0} is the flow rate of tracer from the environment to compartment i; f_{0i} the flow rate from compartment i to the environment and f_{ij} the flow rate from compartment j to compartment i. Here, x_i, x_i^0, f_{i0}, f_{0i} and f_{ij} are all non-negative.

In the compartmental model, the flow between compartments depends on the amount of tracer in the donor compartment but is independent of the quantity in the acceptor compartment. The rate constants f_{ij} and f_{0j} also depend on time t, i.e., time variant.

Introducing the vector notations, $x = (x_1, x_2, \cdots, x_n)^T$, $F = (f_1, f_2, \cdots, f_n)^T$, and $u = [f_{10}, \cdots, f_{n0}]^T$, Eq. 1 is rewritten as

$$\begin{cases} \dot{x} = F(x, t) + u \\ x(0) = x^0, \end{cases} \qquad (2)$$

where $f_i = \sum_{j \neq i} f_{ij} - \left(\sum_{j \neq i} f_{ji} + f_{0i}\right)$.

The system described by Eq. 2 is defined as the compartmental system.

2.2 LINEAR COMPARTMENTAL SYSTEM

When the flow rate f_{ij} from compartment j to compartment i is proportional to x_j but independent of time, f_{ij} is written as

$$f_{ij} = k_{ij} x_j \quad (i, j = 1, \cdots, n, \quad i \neq j), \tag{3}$$

where k_{ij} is the rate constant of the tracer from compartment j to compartment i.

Eq. 2 can then be reduced to:

$$\begin{cases} \dot{x} = Ax + u \\ x(0) = x^0, \end{cases} \tag{4}$$

where the element of the matrix $A = \{a_{ij}\}$ is defined as

$$\begin{cases} a_{ij} = k_{ij} \quad (i \neq j) \\ a_{ii} = -k_{0i} - \sum_{j \neq i} k_{ji}. \end{cases} \tag{5}$$

The system represented by Eq. 4 is a linear compartmental system. The matrix A is called a compartmental matrix. The simplicity of this linear compartmental model permits its broad application in tracer kinetic studies.

If the observations are made at equal sampling intervals τ in Eq. 4, the time-discrete model of the compartmental system is written as

$$\begin{cases} x(n+1) = e^{A\tau} x(n) + \int_0^\tau e^{At} dt \cdot u(n) \\ x(0) = x^0 \end{cases} \tag{6}$$

or

$$\begin{cases} x(n+1) = (I + \tau A) x(n) + \tau \cdot u(n) \\ x(0) = x^0. \end{cases} \tag{6}'$$

This representation is frequently used in medicine because medical data are often taken with time-discrete sampling. This time-discrete model is also applicable to epidemiology, e.g., analysis of follow-up data in chronic diseases.

2.3 HISTORICAL PERSPECTIVE

The use of models resembling compartmental models to represent a system, dates back to Fourier who, in the first half of the 19th century, derived the differential equation based on the continuity of the flow of a substance. The next important step was the introduction of tracer substances to clinical medicine and research. The earliest studies using tracers included estimates of cardiac output (Fick in the second half of the 19th century; Hamilton early in the 20th century.)[5] Teorell (1937) used a two-compartment model to represent the pharmacokinetics involved in a biological system[6]. Tracer kinetic studies advanced rapidly when radioisotopes become available in the 1950's The term compartmental analysis may have been introduced by Sheppard in 1948[7].

Tracer experiments also encouraged the development of mathematical theory in compartmental analysis. This development was accelerated by the introduction of computers to medicine and biology in the 1960's; for example, Perl (1960) reported a method of identification of parameters in a compartmental system[8]. Today, compartmental analysis is widely used for tracer kinetic studies.

3. APPLICATION OF COMPARTMENTAL SYSTEMS

Based on the principle that the simplest possible explanation is preferred, compartmental modeling is applied when the assumptions drawn logically fit the objectives of a problem. In medicine, tests of physiological function, such as the radiocardiogram, radiorenogram, radioencephalogram, and the PSP test, in which a radioisotope or dye is administered, are frequently analyzed by the compartmental model. This model is also used to evaluate fluid and electrolyte balance. Pharmacokinetic studies are almost entirely based on the compartmental model, which is also applicable in epidemiology, assuming that the states of illness, i.e., classifications of severity of disease, are compartments and the number of patients is the amount of tracer. Examples of the application of compartmental analysis to the various fields of medicine are presented in Part II.

In addition to medical applications, compartmental analysis provides a means for analyzing tracer kinetics in a variety of fields, including ecology, economy, and education. Additional fields are given in Table 1.

Table 1. Fields, excluding medicine, in which compartmental analysis can be applied

Field	Compartment	State variable
Ecology	class of age, occupying space, species	population size, population size, population size
Economics	type of industry, region	goods, goods
Business	firm	number of equipment
Administration	hierarchy	number of employees
Pedagogics	grade achieved	population of students

4. THEORETICAL PROBLEMS OF COMPARTMENTAL ANALYSIS

Since the compartmental model describes the flow of substances, their input, output, state variables, and rate constants are all non-negative. This type of system therefore is called a positive system in terms of the dynamic system theory. As a positive system, the compartmental model has several important properties, e.g., the possible region for eigen-values of the compartmental matrix has a special restriction in a complex plane. Accordingly, theoretical considerations relative to the system are important for the practical application of compartmental analysis. Problems include the following:

1. *System identification*
   (a) Identification of transfer function
   (b) Estimation of rate constants
   (c) Estimation of the number of compartments
   (e) Optimal sampling condition
   (f) Identifiability
   (g) Realizability
2. *System Analysis*
   (a) Reachability
   (b) Controllability
   (c) Observability
   (d) Relation between system structure and final state
3. *System Control*
   (a) Optimal control

Although some of the problems remain unsolved in general and complete forms, important findings have been made in the linear time invariant compartmental system in which the compartmental matrix A in Eq. 4 is independent of time. For example, recent advances are apparent in the study of identifiability. Structural identifiability implies that transition coefficients (rate constants) can be derived from the transfer function when the structure of the model and the sites of input and output are known. Conversely, transition coefficients cannot be determined from input-output responses, if the system is not "structurally identifiable." Accordingly, structure identifiability should be tested, along with practical applications of compartmental analysis. Important findings related to system theory are presented in Part 1.

Finally, the reader need not start to read this book from its beginning, following the sequence given in the Contents. Anyone interested in compartmental analysis can open this book at any chapter, as each has been written rather independently, keeping in mind the relevancy of topics in each chapter.

REFERENCES

1 Atkins, G.L.: *Multicompartment Models for Biological Systems*. Muthuen, London, 1969.
2 Jacquez, J.A.: *Compartmental Analysis in Biology and Medicine*. Elsevier, New York, 1972.
3 Watt, K.E.F.: *System Analysis in Ecology*. Academic Press, New York, 1973.
4 Brown, R.F.: Compartmental system analysis: State of Art. *IEEE Trans*. BME-27: 1-11, 1980.
5 Zierler, K.: A critique of compartmental analysis. *Ann. Rev. Biophys. Bioeng.* 10: 531-562, 1981.
6 Teorell, T.: Kinetics of distribution of substances administered to the body. I. The extravascular modes of administration. *Arch. Int. Pharmacodyn. Ther.* 57: 205-225, 1937. II. The intravascular modes of administration. *Arch. Int. Pharmacodyn. Ther.* 57: 226-240, 1937.
7 Sheppard, C.W.: The theory of the study of transfers within a multi-compartmental system using isotopic tracers. *J.Appl. Phys.* 19: 70-76, 1948.
8 Perl, W.: A method for curve-fitting by exponential functions. *Int. J. Appl. Radiat. Isotop.* 8: 211-222, 1960.

PART ONE

1
ESTIMATION OF PARAMETERS IN COMPARTMENTAL ANALYSIS

Fumihiko Kajiya, Mitsuyasu Kagiyama, Noritake Hoki and Kyoji Kawagoe

1. INTRODUCTION

Compartmental analysis is a method whereby a system composed of several compartments is evaluated by observing the dynamics of a tracer substance introduced into the system.

In terms of system theory, the linear compartmental system can be represented by the following dynamic equation,

$$\dot{x}_i(t) = -\left(a_{0i} + \sum_{j \neq i}^{p} a_{ji}\right) x_i(t) + \sum_{j \neq i}^{p} a_{ij} x_j(t) + b_i(t), \tag{1}$$

where x_i is the amount or concentration of tracer in the ith compartment, p is the number of compartments, $a_{ij}(i \neq j)$ the rate constant from the jth to the ith compartment, a_{0i} the rate constant at which tracer is lost from the ith compartment to the outside of the system, and b_i is the input (Fig. 1).

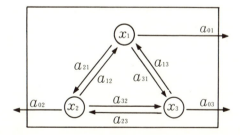

Fig. 1. Three-compartment model and its rate constants.

Defining $-\left(a_{0i}+\sum_{j\neq i}^{p}a_{ji}\right)=a_{ii}$, we have

$$\dot{x}_i(t)=\sum_{j=1}^{p}a_{ij}x_j(t)+b_i(t). \qquad (2)$$

From the physical characteristics of the compartmental system, e.g., the law "constancy of tracer mass", this system has the following properties[1,2]:

(i) $a_{ij}\geq 0$, $i\neq j$, $a_{ii}\leq 0$,
(ii) $|a_{jj}|\geq \sum_{i\neq j}a_{ij}$. $\qquad (3)$

The identification problem in compartmental analysis is to estimate a_{ij} in Eq. 1 or Eq. 2 from the input-output data of a tracer under the constraints of Eq. 3. In practice the problem of identification is classified into (a) type-1, the number of compartments is not given before identification[3-6], and (b) type-2, the structure of the compartmental system, i.e., the number of compartments and their combination, is given beforehand[7].

For the type-1 problem, a general solution is impossible. However, in special types of compartmental models, such as the catenary and mamillary models, the dynamic behavior of the tracer is theoretically shown to follow the sum of exponential functions[17],

$$y(t)=\sum_{i=1}^{p}A_i e^{-a_i t}, \qquad (4)$$

where A_i and a_i ($i=1,\cdots,p$) are real numbers. The first step considered in this type of problem is the estimation of (a) the number of compartment p as well as (b) the pertinent parameters A_i and a_i. Many attempts have been made to develop adequate means to estimate parameters in multi-exponential functions. They include the methods: (a) peeling[8], (b) moments[9], (c) least squares estimation[10], (d) maximum likelihood[11], (e) Fourier transform[12,13], and (f) Prony's[14]. In practical application, however, the estimation of the number of compartments is crucial, owing to the inevitable presence of noise in the data.

We have demonstrated that an information theoretical criterion (AIC), introduced by Akaike[15,16], can be successfully applied in most cases to the estimation of p.

When the object of analysis is a medical or biological system, the tracer is frequently a radioisotope. Radioisotope (RI) data can be modelled by a Poisson process with a count rate dependent variance[17,18]. In this chapter the observation is considered to obey a Poisson distribution. For the estimation of A_i and a_i, the maximum likelihood method[17] was used because it is a consistent means of estimation when the likelihood function can be defined, as in RI tracer kinetic data.

In the first part of this chapter, the maximum likelihood method combined with AIC is described for the estimation of A_i, a_i, and p.

The method of estimating exponential functions in compartmental analysis, however, cannot be applied to a system such as the cyclical compartmental system, because the exponential terms will have some imaginary parts. Under these conditions, it is necessary to estimate $\{a_{ij}\}$, in Eq. 2, directly from the input-output data. This belongs to the type-2 problem.

In the latter section of this chapter, the method for estimating the parameters when the structure of the compartmental system, i.e., the number of compartments and their combination, are given beforehand is described.

2. ESTIMATION OF PARAMETERS WHEN THE DYNAMIC BEHAVIOR OF THE TRACER FOLLOWS THE SUM OF EXPONENTIAL FUNCTIONS[3-6]

This section presents a method of estimating exponential functions for RI tracer kinetic data after the impulse input of tracer. AIC and the maximum likelihood method were applied to estimate parameters in exponential functions.

The RI value read at time t_j is written by the time integral of the count during the sampling interval $t_{j-1} - t_j$, i.e.,

$$\text{RI count} = \int_{t_{j-1}}^{t_j} \sum A_i e^{-a_i t} dt. \tag{5}$$

For simplicity, in this section the mean value function $\langle n_j \rangle$ of the output at time t_j can be expressed as,

$$\langle n_j \rangle = \sum A_i e^{-a_i t}, \tag{6}$$

since it is easy to generalize the expression of Eq. 6 to that of Eq. 5.

2.1 METHODS

Assume that there are m independent observations $n_1, n_2, \cdots, n_m$. Since the probability of the value n_j in the jth observation is assumed to be Poissonian, $P(n_j; \theta_1, \theta_2, \cdots, \theta_{2p}) = \exp(-\langle n_j \rangle)(\langle n_j \rangle^{n_j}/n_j!)$, the joint probability corresponding to the likelihood function L can be written as

$$L = \prod_{j=1}^{m} P(n_j; \theta_1, \theta_2, \cdots, \theta_{2p})$$
$$= \exp\left(-\sum_{j=1}^{m} \langle n_j \rangle\right) \frac{\langle n_1 \rangle^{n_1} \langle n_2 \rangle^{n_2} \cdots \langle n_m \rangle^{n_m}}{n_1! n_2! \cdots n_m!}, \qquad (7)$$

where $\langle n_j \rangle$ is the expected value of $\sum_{i=1}^{p} A_i e^{-\alpha_i t_j}$ and parameters $\{(\theta_1, \cdots, \theta_p)(\theta_{p+1}, \cdots, \theta_{2p})\}$ represent $(A_1, A_2, \cdots, A_p)$ and $(\alpha_1, \alpha_2, \cdots, \alpha_p)$, respectively.

Taking the logarithm of Eq. 7 and applying Stirling formula $[k! \cong \sqrt{2\pi k} \cdot k^k \exp(-k)]$, we have

$$\ln L = -\sum_{j=1}^{m} \{\langle n_j \rangle - n_j \ln \langle n_j \rangle + n_j \ln(n_j) - n_j + 1/2 \ln(2\pi n_j)\}. \qquad (8)$$

The problem then is to estimate the $2p$ parameters $(A_1, \cdots, A_p)$ and $(\alpha_1, \cdots, \alpha_p)$ so as to minimize $-\ln L$. For this nonlinear optimization problem, the simplex method of Nelder and Mead[19] was applied because it can create its own scaling factor and converges for a wide range of starting points.

For the estimation of p, AIC[15,16] defined as

$$\text{AIC}(_k\hat{\theta}) = -2 \sum_{i=1}^{m} \ln f(n_i/_k\hat{\theta}) + 2k \qquad (9)$$

was applied in which k is the number of independently adjustable parameters within the model and $_k\hat{\theta}$ is the vector of the maximum likelihood estimates of $_k\theta = (\theta_1 \cdots, \theta_k)$. The number k of the model corresponding to the minimum AIC is selected as the optimal one. This criterion represents a measure of the fitness of a model to given statistical data and has been successfully applied for statistical model identification problems in a wide range of fields. Since there are $2p$ parameters in our case, k in Eq. 9 is replaced by $2p$, and

$$\text{AIC} = -2 \ln(\text{maximum likelihood}) + 4p. \qquad (10)$$

Thus the estimation scheme is the following: Step 1 — start with $p = 1$. Estimate the A_i and α_i for a given p by the maximum likelihood method. Step 2 — evaluate AIC using the results obtained in Step 1. Step 3 — repeat step 1 and step 2 for $p = 1, 2, 3 \cdots$. Find the value of p that minimizes AIC. This p and the corresponding A_i and α_i are used as our estimation.

2.2 APPLICATION TO EXPONENTIAL DATA

Compartmental analysis is usually carried out for up to three exponential terms. Consequently, to investigate the effects of the number of exponentials and of sample size on estimates of A_i, a_i and p, the following mean value functions with Poisson distribution were used as test functions:

$$y_1(t) = 100e^{-0.01t},$$
$$y_2(t) = 100e^{-0.01t} + 200e^{-0.05t},$$
$$y_3(t) = 100e^{-0.01t} + 200e^{-0.05t} + 300e^{-0.2t}.$$

Estimations were performed for three different sample sizes ($m=50$, 100 and 200) with a fixed sampling interval ($\tau=1$). The results are given in Table 1. Note that irrespective of the sample size, the minimum AIC values for $y_1(t)$ and $y_2(t)$ correctly indicate the number of exponentials contained in the test functions. This is also true for $y_3(t)$, when $m=100$ or 200 is used; for $m=50$, however, the number is underestimated as 2. Then the asymptotic variance of each parameter for $y_3(t)$ was calculated theoretically, according to the method described in the next chapter (Table 2). The results suggest that the values of asymptotic variances for $m=50$ are too large to identify the number of p.

The accuracy of the estimations of A_i and a_i in $y_1(t)$ and $y_2(t)$ is reasonably good, even when the sample size is small. But the accuracy of estimates for $y_3(t)$ changes with the sample size; the errors of estimates with $m=100$ are over 50 percent, while with $m=200$, they are within 10%.

To test the resolution of the present method, the following mean value functions, with two similar decay constants, were chosen as test functions:

$$y_4(t) = 100e^{-0.01t} + 200e^{-0.015t},$$
$$y_5(t) = 100e^{-0.05t} + 200e^{-0.1t},$$
$$y_6(t) = 100e^{-0.05t} + 200e^{-0.075t}.$$

Estimates were made with two different sampling intervals ($\tau=1, 5$; $m=200$) for $y_4(t)$ and with three different sample sizes ($m=50, 100, 200$; $\tau=1$) for $y_5(t)$ and $y_6(t)$. The results are shown in Table 3. Note that correct estimates for p are obtained in all cases except for $y_4(t)$, in which p is underestimated as 1 when $\tau=1$ and $m=200$ are used, and also for $y_5(t)$, in which p is similarly underestimated as 1 with $m=50$ and $\tau=1$.

To elucidate a critical efficacy in the resolution of exponentials by the

Table 1. Effect of sample size and number of exponentials on estimation of A_i, α_i and p (Underline indicates the minimum AIC values for various assumed orders) : Sampling interval $\tau = 1$

$$Y_1(t) = 100e^{-0.01t}$$

Order Sample size	1	2 (1/2 AIC values)	3	4	Estimation of each parameter
50	<u>181.1</u>	182.7	184.6	186.7	$102.7e^{-0.0099t}$
100	<u>345.8</u>	347.6	349.6	351.9	$103.3e^{-0.0102t}$
200	<u>631.7</u>	633.5	635.7	637.7	$103.1e^{-0.0101t}$

$$Y_2(t) = 100e^{-0.01t} + 200e^{-0.05t}$$

Order Sample size	1	2 (1/2 AIC values)	3	4	Estimation of each parameter
50	205.1	<u>201.6</u>	203.6	205.6	$105e^{-0.0093t} + 205e^{-0.0523t}$
100	426.9	<u>371.2</u>	373.0	375.0	$93e^{-0.0089t} + 215e^{-0.0484t}$
200	891.8	<u>656.6</u>	658.2	660.2	$97e^{-0.0096t} + 210e^{-0.0483t}$

$$Y_3(t) = 100e^{-0.01t} + 200e^{-0.05t} + 300e^{-0.2t}$$

Order Sample size	1	2 (1/2 AIC values)	3	4	Estimation of each parameter
50	333.7	<u>200.6</u>	205.7	207.3	$234e^{-0.0219t} + 382e^{-0.175t}$
100	761.1	379.3	<u>375.1</u>	377.1	$40e^{-0.0162t} + 240e^{-0.035t} + 341e^{-0.193t}$
200	1496.5	680.1	<u>665.9</u>	673.3	$108e^{-0.0104t} + 219e^{-0.054t} + 297e^{-0.218t}$

Table 2. The Asymptotic variances of A_i and α_i in $y_3(t) = 100e^{-0.01t} + 200e^{-0.05t} + 300e^{-0.2t}$ at sample size 50, 100, and 200 (Figures in parentheses are square roots of variances)

Parameter Sample size	$\alpha_1 = 0.01$	$\alpha_2 = 0.05$	$\alpha_3 = 0.2$	$A_1 = 100$	$A_2 = 200$	$A_3 = 300$
50	0.33×10^{-1} (0.182)	0.141 (0.375)	0.30×10^{-1} (0.173)	0.241×10^7 (1552)	0.119×10^7 (1091)	0.226×10^6 (475)
100	0.63×10^{-4} (0.79×10^{-2})	0.13×10^{-2} (0.36×10^{-1})	0.34×10^{-2} (0.58×10^{-1})	7682 (87.6)	2090 (45.7)	9142 (95.6)
200	0.74×10^{-6} (0.86×10^{-3})	0.12×10^{-3} (0.11×10^{-1})	0.15×10^{-2} (0.39×10^{-1})	175.9 (13.3)	1685.3 (41.1)	2196.3 (46.9)

Table 3. Effect of a pair of similar exponential terms

$$Y_4(t) = 100e^{-0.01t} + 200e^{-0.015t}$$

Order Sampling interval	1	2 (1/2 AIC value)	3	4	Estimation of each parameter
$\tau=1.0$	<u>724.9</u>	736.3	727.8	730.3	$305e^{-0.013t}$
$\tau=5.0$	309.9	<u>302.2</u>	308.8	310.1	$213e^{-0.011t} + 102e^{-0.021t}$

$$Y_5(t) = 100e^{-0.05t} + 200e^{-0.01t}$$

Order Sample size	1	2 (1/2 AIC value)	3	4	Estimation of each parameter
50	174.5	<u>167.4</u>	169.4	171.5	$35e^{-0.0267t} + 277e^{-0.0921t}$
100	267.6	<u>251.8</u>	253.7	255.6	$138e^{-0.0533t} + 175e^{-0.115t}$
200	310.0	<u>287.5</u>	289.3	290.7	$117e^{-0.0510t} + 195e^{-0.107t}$

$$Y_6(t) = 100e^{-0.05t} + 200e^{-0.075t}$$

Order Sample size	1	2 (1/2 AIC value)	3	4	Estimation of each parameter
50	<u>177.7</u>	179.4	181.4	182.6	$307e^{-0.0647t}$
100	283.2	<u>279.1</u>	281.4	283.0	$79e^{-0.0444t} + 234e^{-0.0772t}$
200	310.0	<u>307.2</u>	309.2	313.2	$102e^{-0.103t} + 213e^{-0.0557t}$

present method, $y_5(t)$ and $y_6(t)$ are noted. The rates of the first and second decay constants for $y_5(t)$ is $1/2$; the ratio for $y_6(t)$ is $2/3$. As stated earlier, $y_5(t)$ is estimated correctly, whereas p is underestimated in $y_6(t)$ with $m=50$. Then the asymptotic variance of each parameter in $y_5(t)$, and $y_6(t)$ was calculated by the method described in the next chapter (Table 4). Comparison of the asymptotic variances of both functions shows that values in $y_5(t)$ are much smaller than those in $y_6(t)$. These results indicate that asymptotic variance is one of the important factors in the evaluation of a critical resolution of exponentials by the present method.

2.3 CONCLUDING REMARKS

To estimate the number of compartments p, AIC was applied because it is a versatile procedure applicable to every situation in which likelihood can be defined. It also provides a model of identification without subjective judgment. The results of estimating p by AIC correlated well with the number of exponentials in the test functions, except in cases with large

Table 4. Asymptotic variance of A_i and α_i for functions with similar exponential terms (Figures in parentheses are square roots of the variances)

$Y_5(t)$

Sample size	Parameter			
	$\alpha_1=0.05$	$\alpha_2=0.1$	$A_1=100$	$A_2=200$
50	0.15×10^{-2} (0.39×10^{-1})	0.29×10^{-2} (0.54×10^{-1})	60496 (246)	57813 (240)
100	0.68×10^{-4} (0.82×10^{-2})	0.40×10^{-2} (0.63×10^{-1})	4158 (64)	3684 (61)
200	0.24×10^{-4} (0.49×10^{-2})	0.20×10^{-3} (0.14×10^{-1})	1743 (42)	1512 (39)

$Y_6(t)$

Sample size	Parameter			
	$\alpha_1=0.05$	$\alpha_2=0.075$	$A_1=100$	$A_2=200$
50	0.26×10^{-1} (0.161)	0.19×10^{-1} (0.138)	0.277×10^7 (1664)	0.275×10^7 (1658)
100	0.77×10^{-3} (0.28×10^{-1})	0.11×10^{-2} (0.33×10^{-1})	0.11×10^6 (332)	0.107×10^6 (327)
200	0.15×10^{-3} (0.12×10^{-1})	0.33×10^{-3} (0.18×10^{-1})	25303 (159)	24153 (155)

asymptotic variances.

As mentioned in the Introduction and in the section on Methods, the observations are assumed to obey a Poisson distribution and are independent over time. Under these assumptions, the maximum likelihood method can provide an optimal estimate of A_i, and α_i in that the likelihood function tends to be a most sensitive criterion of the deviation of model parameters from true values. Sander et al.[11] developed maximum likelihood in the analysis of tracer kinetics and demonstrated its usefulness. This method leads to the nonlinear optimization problem, as shown in Eq. 8. We have applied the simplex method of Nelder and Mead, since it can create its own scaling factor and converges for a wide range of starting points. The final points of convergence agreed with the given set of values for each parameter.

In conclusion, it is both feasible and useful to apply AIC, and the maximum likelihood method, to the identification of multiexponential functions in RI tracer kinetic data.

3. IDENTIFICATION OF PARAMETERS IN A COMPARTMENTAL SYSTEM WHEN THE STRUCTURE IS GIVEN BEFOREHAND[7]

In the previous section we discussed the maximum likelihood method combined with AIC to estimate pertinent parameters in exponential functions from RI kinetic data. In practice, however, there are some cases in which the output cannot be expressed by multiexponential functions with real exponential parts, as in a cyclical system.

A method is presented that can be used to identify a_{ij} in Eq. 2 from input-output data, when the structure — i.e., the number of compartments and their combination is known *apriori* from medical experiences. This method is applicable when observations cannot be expressed by multi-exponential functions.

The output, i.e., RI count in this section, is considered to be represented by the time integral of the count during the sampling interval.

3. 1 METHODS
3. 1. 1 Description of the problem

We suppose that there are r observations from r compartments at time t_j; $n(t_j) = \{n_1(t_j), \cdots, n_r(t_j)\}$, $j=1, 2, \cdots, m$. Since the RI count at t_j is the time integral between t_{j-1} and t_j, the expected value $\langle n_k(t_j) \rangle$ of $n(t_j)$ is written as:

$$\langle n_k(t_j) \rangle = \int_{t_{j-1}}^{t_j} x_k(t) dt, \quad k=1, 2, \cdots, r. \tag{11}$$

As mentioned in the previous section, RI data obey a Poisson distribution. Thus, the likelihood function for $n(t_j)$, $j=1, \cdots, m$ is given by:[1]

$$L = \prod_{k=1}^{r} e^{-\sum_{j=1}^{m} \langle n_k(t_j) \rangle} \cdot \frac{\langle n_k(t_1) \rangle^{n_k(t_1)} \langle n_k(t_2) \rangle^{n_k(t_2)} \cdots \langle n_k(t_m) \rangle^{n_k(t_m)}}{n_k(t_1)! \, n_k(t_2)! \cdots n_k(t_m)!}. \tag{12}$$

Taking the logarithm of Eq. 12, we have

$$\ln L = -\sum_{k=1}^{r}\sum_{j=1}^{m} (\langle n_k(t_j) \rangle - n_k(t_j) \ln \langle n_k(t_j) \rangle + \ln n_k(t_j)!). \tag{13}$$

This can be approximated as Eq. 14 by applying the Starling formula:

$$\ln L \cong -\sum_{k=1}^{r}\sum_{j=1}^{m} \left(\langle n_k(t_j) \rangle - n_k(t_j) - n_k(t_j) \ln \frac{\langle n_k(t_j) \rangle}{n_k(t_j)} \right). \tag{14}$$

Since $|\langle n_k(t_j) \rangle - n_k(t_j)|$ is considered to be much smaller than $n_k(t_j)$, i.e.,

$\dfrac{|\langle n_k(t_j)\rangle - n_k(t_j)|}{n_k(t_j)} \ll 1$, the third term of the right hand side of Eq. 14 is approximated as:

$$n_k(t_j)\ln\dfrac{\langle n_k(t_j)\rangle}{n_k(t_j)} = n_k(t_j)\ln\left(1+\dfrac{\langle n_k(t_j)\rangle - n_k(t_j)}{n_k(t_j)}\right)$$

$$\cong n_k(t_j)\left\{\dfrac{\langle n_k(t_j)\rangle - n_k(t_j)}{n_k(t_j)} - \dfrac{(\langle n_k(t_j)\rangle - n_k(t_j))^2}{2n_k(t_j)^2}\right\}$$

$$= \langle n_k(t_j)\rangle - n_k(t_j) - \dfrac{1}{2}\dfrac{(\langle n_k(t_j)\rangle - n_k(t_j))^2}{n_k(t_j)}. \quad (15)$$

Then Eq. 14 can be approximated as

$$\ln L \cong -\dfrac{1}{2}\sum_{k=1}^{r}\sum_{j=1}^{m}\dfrac{(\langle n_k(t_j)\rangle - n_k(t_j))^2}{n_k(t_j)}. \quad (16)$$

In the following, "$-2\ln L$" is defined as "J," that is the sum of squares of the residuals weighted by the reciprocal of the observed values.

Now, the problem is to minimize "J" under the following constraints:
1. The state variable x is the solution of Eq. 2.
2. The rate constants $\{a_{ij}\}$ satisfy the inequalities in Eq. 3.

3.1.2 Optimization

To remove constraint (2), the following transformation was made:

$$\begin{cases} a_{ij} = c_{ij}^2 & (i \neq j), \\ a_{ii} = -\sum_{k \neq i} c_{ik}^2 - c_{ii}^2. \end{cases} \quad (17)$$

The problem now becomes an ordinary nonlinear optimization for the parameter $\{c_{ij}\}$ without constraints. For this nonlinear optimization, the simplex method of Nelder and Mead[18] was again used for the same reason as in the previous section.

3.2 ESTIMATION IN MODEL COMPARTMENTS

To investigate the accuracy of estimates obtained by the present method, two types of compartmental systems were used as the test model (Fig. 2). For ease of evaluation, it was assumed that an impulse input is applied to one compartment and observations are made for that compartment. Since the output of model A can be represented by the sum of two real exponential functions, the method mentioned in the previous section will also be applicable to estimates of the parameter. However, note that the output function of model B will have imaginary exponential parts, in which the rate constants a_{ij} must be estimated directly from observation data.

The outputs were superimposed with Poisson fluctuation for the simulation of RI data. The estimates were made for several different sampling intervals, with a fixed sample size ($\tau = 50$). Each experiment was repeated 5 times by varying the initial values of random numbers to generate Poisson fluctuation, and standard deviations (SD) were calculated. The asymptotic variances (see the next chapter) were also calculated and compared with the standard errors.

3.3 RESULTS AND CONCLUDING REMARKS

Parameter values were chosen as $a_{21}=0.1$, $a_{12}=0.05$, $a_{01}=0.1$ and $b=500$ in model A, and $a_{21}=0.08$, $a_{32}=0.03$, $a_{13}=0.1$, $a_{01}=0.02$ and $b=800$ in model B. The estimated values for models A and B are shown in Figure 3; sampling intervals are plotted along the horizontal axes and values for parameters along the vertical axes. Open circles represent the mean value of each estimate. The horizontal lines represent the true (given) value of each parameter while vertical bars represent 2 standard deviations (SD). Downward and upward convex curves represent twice the values of asymptotic variances ($\hat{\sigma}$) obtained theoretically.

In models A and B the accuracy of estimated values for a_{ij} by the present method is reasonably good, as the mean value of each estimate (open circles) agrees well with the true (preset) value, except under sampling conditions with large asymptotic variances.

Although the number of repetitions for estimating standard deviations is small, changes in 2 SD with sampling intervals show a trend similar to the $2\hat{\sigma}$ curves; the ranges of ± 2SD lie almost within $\pm 2\hat{\sigma}$. These results

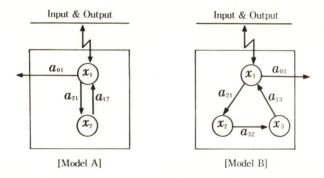

Fig. 2. Two- and 3-compartment models used for numerical experiments.

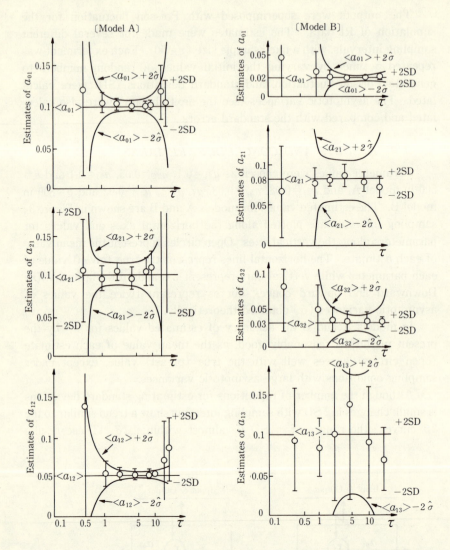

Fig. 3. Mean values, standard deviations and asymptotic variances of estimated parameters (Model A and Model B) for each sampling interval (abscissa). Open circles represent mean values, vertical bars standard deviations (2SD), downward and upward convex curves asymptotic variances ($2\hat{\sigma}$).

indicate that asymptotic variance provides a good estimate of the variance of parameters in the maximum likelihood method. It should be noted that an optimal sampling interval exists which minimizes the asymptotic variances for all parameters, both in model A and in model B. This interval will be discussed in the next chapter.

In conclusion, the maximum likelihood method was also found useful for estimating the parameter in compartmental analysis when the structure of the compartment is known beforehand.

ACKNOWLEDGMENT

We are grateful to the IEEE for permission to partly reproduce our paper published in IEEE Trans. BME-26 (7) : 422-427, 1979.

REFERENCES

1. Sheppard, C.W. & Hauseholder, A.S.: The mathematical basis of the interpretation of tracer experiments in closed steady state systems. *J. Appl. Physiol.* 22 : 510-520, 1951.
2. Hearon, J.Z.: Theorems on linear systems. *Ann. N.Y. Acad. Sci.* 108 : 36-67, 1963.
3. Kajiya, F., Kawagoe, K. & Kodama, S.: A method of study of radioactive tracer kinetics. *IEEE Trans.* BME-26 : 422-428, 1979.
4. Kajiya, F., Hoki, N. & Imamura, M.: Compartmental analysis in radioisotope tracer kinetics —— Identification and the optimal experimental design —— *Proc. of 2nd Int. Symp. on Med. Inform. System* 113-117, 1978.
5. Kajiya, F.: Compartmental Analysis. Thesis, Osaka University, 1977 (in Japanese).
6. Kajiya, F., Kawagoe, K., Maeda, H. et al.: Estimation of the number of compartments and each parameter value in the compartmental analysis. *Trans. IECE* 60-D-3 : 209-215, 1977 (in Japanese).
7. Kagiyama, M., Kajiya, F., Hoki, N. et al.: Identification of parameters in compartmental system when the structure is given beforehand. *Systems Computers Controls* 11 : 82-90, Scripta Publishing Co., New York, 1980.
8. Mancini, P. & Pilo, A.: A computer program for multiexponential fitting by the peeling method. *Comp. Biomed. Res.* 3 : 1-14, 1970.
9. Isenberg, I. & Dyson, R.D.: The analysis of fluorescence decay by a method of moments. *Biophys. J.* 9 : 1337-1350, 1969.
10. Marcquardt, D.W.: An algorithm for least squares estimation of nonlinear parameters. *J. Soc. Indust. Appl. Math.* 11 : 431-441, 1963.
11. Sandor, T., Conroy, M.F. & Hollenberg, N.K.: The application of the method of maximum likelihood to the analysis of tracer kinetic data. *Math. Biosci.* 9 : 149-159, 1970.
12. Kajiya, F., Yamano, Y., Inada, H. et al.: Estimation of the number of compartments and exponential functions in compartment analysis. *Behavior Metrics* 2 : 1-8, 1975 (in Japanese).
13. Garder, D.G.: Resolution of multicomponent exponential decay curves using fourier transforms. *Ann. N.Y. Acad. Sci.* 108 : 195-203, 1963.

14 Hilderbrand, F.B.: *Introduction to Numerical Analysis.* McGraw-Hill Inc. New York, 1956.
15 Akaike, H.: A new look at the statistical model identification. *IEEE Trans.* AC-19: 716-723, 1974.
16 Akaike, H.: Information theory and the statistical model identification. *Math. Biosci.* 9: 37-47, 1970.
17 Shoenfeld, R.L. & Berman, M.: An electrical network analogy for isotope kinetics. *IRE Nat. Conv. Rec.* 4: 84-89, 1957.
18 Wagner, H.N., Jr., Walton, W.W., Jr. & Jacquez, J.: *Mathematics in Principles of Nuclear Medicine.* H.N. Wagner, ed. Toronto, Ont., Canada. Saunders, 1968.
19 Nelder, M.A. & Mead, R.: A simplex method for function minimization. *Comp. J.* 7: 308-313, 1965.

2

OPTIMUM SAMPLING FOR THE IDENTIFICATION OF COMPARTMENTAL SYSTEMS

Fumihiko Kajiya, Mitsuyasu Kagiyama, Masatsugu Hori, Katsuhiko Tsujioka and Go Tomonaga

1. INTRODUCTION

It is widely recognized that compartmental analysis offers a useful mathematical method for the kinetic study of tracers widely used in clinical and basic medicine. However, due to noise included in the observation data, estimations of parameters are not always reliable in a compartmental system. As mentioned in the previous chapter, the accuracy of the estimates is influenced by sampling conditions, i.e., sample size and sampling interval.

This chapter considers the asymptotic variances of parameters in the maximum likelihood estimation. As an approach to such a sampling problem, Bergner and others[1] calculated the unbiased variance for numerical examples in which the noise follows a Gaussian distribution. When the object of analysis is a medical system, however, the tracer is frequently a radioisotope (RI). Accordingly, as in the previous chapter, the tracer is assumed to be a RI, and the observation therefore, obeys a Poisson distribution[2]. The asymptotic variances of parameters are calculated by using Fisher's information and the Cramer-Rao inequality.

The RI count, read at time t_j, is the output obtained by integrating the count in the sampling interval $t_j - t_{j-1}$; the count itself is a function of the sampling interval. The mean value function, $\langle n_i(t_j) \rangle$, of the output from the ith compartment at time t_j is written as

$$\langle n_i(t_j) \rangle = \int_{t_{j-1}}^{t_j} x_i(t) dt, \tag{1}$$

where $x_i(t)$ $(i=1, \cdots, p)$ denotes the state variable (tracer amount) of the compartment.

In the special types of compartmental systems, such as the catenary or mammillary systems, which are frequently used in medical fields, $x_i(t)$ in Eq. 1 is written by the sum of exponential functions as

$$x(t) = \sum_{i=1}^{p} A_i e^{-\alpha_i t}. \qquad (2)$$

This type of situation is considered in the first part of this chapter.

Second, asymptotic variances of estimates are evaluated for cases in which the structure of the compartmental system is given beforehand.

2. EFFECT OF SAMPLING CONDITIONS ON ACCURACY OF IDENTIFICATION FOR MULTIEXPONENTIAL FUNCTIONS[5]

2.1 ASYMPTOTIC VARIANCES OF PARAMETERS

Assume that m independent observations $n_1, n_2, \cdots, n_m$ are made in a system containing $2p$ parameters $\theta_1, \theta_2, \cdots, \theta_{2p}$ ($\equiv \alpha_1, \cdots, \alpha_p, A_1, \cdots, A_p$). Let the probability that the jth observed value is n_j be given by $P(n_j : \theta_1, \theta_2, \cdots, \theta_{2p})$. Then the likelihood function L for the observation vector $(n_1, \cdots, n_m)$, can be represented as

$$L = \prod_{j=1}^{m} P(n_j; \theta_1, \cdots, \theta_{2p}). \qquad (3)$$

Introducing the information defined by Fisher[3], the (k, l) element I_{kl} of the information matrix I is given by the expression:

$$I_{kl} = E\left\{ \frac{\partial}{\partial \theta_k}(\ln L) \frac{\partial}{\partial \theta_l}(\ln L) \right\}$$
$$= -E\left\{ \frac{\partial^2}{\partial \theta_k \partial \theta_l}(\ln L) \right\}, \qquad (4)$$

where $E\{\cdot\}$ represents the expectation.

Since the Cramer-Rao inequality is valid for multivariable parameters, letting V be the variance-covariance matrix of the unbiased estimates, $\hat{\theta}_1, \hat{\theta}_2, \cdots, \hat{\theta}_m$, $V - I^{-1}$ is non-negative definite[4]. Consequently, for a large sample the diagonal of I^{-1} provides the asymptotic variances of parameters in the maximum likelihood estimation.

When the observation obeys a Poisson distribution, as with a RI tracer, the probability that the observed value at time t_j is n_j is given by

$$P(n_j: \theta_1, \cdots, \theta_{2p}) = e^{-\langle n_j \rangle} \frac{\langle n_j \rangle^{n_j}}{n_j!}. \tag{5}$$

Then, the likelihood function for the observation vector is given by

$$L = e^{-\Sigma \langle n_j \rangle} \frac{\langle n_1 \rangle^{n_1} \langle n_2 \rangle^{n_2} \cdots \langle n_m \rangle^{n_m}}{n_1! \, n_2! \cdots n_m!}. \tag{6}$$

Taking the logarithm of Eq. 6, it follows that

$$\ln L = -\sum_{j=1}^{m} \{\langle n_j \rangle - n_j \ln \langle n_j \rangle + \ln n_j!\}. \tag{7}$$

Consequently, the (k, l) element I_{kl} of the Fisher's information matrix I is written as

$$I_{kl} = -E\left\{\frac{\partial^2}{\partial \theta_k \partial \theta_l}(\Sigma \langle n_j \rangle - \Sigma n_j \ln \langle n_i \rangle)\right\}$$

$$= \sum_{j=1}^{m} \left(\frac{1}{\langle n_j \rangle} \cdot \frac{\partial \langle n_j \rangle}{\partial \theta_k} \cdot \frac{\partial \langle n_j \rangle}{\partial \theta_l}\right). \tag{8}$$

Since the number of counts is the time integral between t_{j-1} and t_j, the count expectation $\langle n_j \rangle$ is given by

$$\langle n_j \rangle = \int_{t_{j-1}}^{t_j} \sum_{i=1}^{p} A_i e^{-a_j t} dt$$

$$= \sum_{i=1}^{p} \frac{A_i}{a_i}(e^{a_i \tau} - 1) e^{-a_i \tau \times j}, \tag{9}$$

where τ is the sampling interval and $t_j = (j-1)\tau$, $j = 1, 2, \cdots, m$.

Then, $\partial \langle n_j \rangle / \partial a_i$ and $\partial \langle n_j \rangle / \partial A_i$ are calculated as

$$\frac{\partial \langle n_j \rangle}{\partial a_i} = -\frac{e^{-a_i j \tau}}{a_i}\left[\frac{1}{a_i}(e^{a_i \tau} - 1) + \tau\{j(e^{a_i \tau} - 1) - e^{a_i \tau}\}\right] A_i, \tag{10}$$

$$\frac{\partial \langle n_j \rangle}{\partial A_i} = -\frac{1}{a_i} e^{-a_i j \tau}(e^{a_i \tau} - 1). \tag{11}$$

As was previously described, the parameter is defined as follows:

$$\theta_i = \begin{cases} a_i, & 1 \leq i \leq p \\ A_{i-p}, & p+1 \leq i \leq 2p. \end{cases}$$

Dividing the Fisher's information matrix I into blocks,

$$I = \begin{bmatrix} \overbrace{I^{(1,1)}}^{p} & \overbrace{I^{(1,2)}}^{p} \\ \hline I^{(2,1)} & I^{(2,2)} \end{bmatrix} \begin{matrix} \}p, \\ \}p \end{matrix}$$

the (k, l) element of each block is calculated as follows, using Eqs. 8, 10 and 11:

$$I_{kl}^{(1,1)} = \sum_{j=1}^{m} \left\{ \frac{1}{\langle n_j \rangle} \cdot \frac{e^{-(\alpha_k+\alpha_l)j\tau}}{\alpha_k \alpha_l} \cdot r_{k,j} \cdot r_{l,j} \right\}, \tag{12}$$

$$I_{kl}^{(2,2)} = \sum_{j=1}^{m} \left\{ \frac{1}{\langle n_j \rangle} \cdot \frac{e^{-(\alpha_k+\alpha_l)j\tau}}{\alpha_k \alpha_l} \cdot (e^{\alpha_k\tau}-1)(e^{\alpha_l\tau}-1) \right\}, \tag{13}$$

$$I_{kl}^{(1,2)} = I_{lk}^{(2,1)} = \sum_{j=1}^{m} \left\{ \frac{-1}{\langle n_j \rangle} \cdot \frac{e^{-(\alpha_k+\alpha_l)j\tau}}{\alpha_k \alpha_l} \cdot (e^{\alpha_l\tau}-1) r_{k,j} \right\}, \tag{14}$$

where $r_{k,j} = \left[\frac{1}{\alpha_k}(e^{\alpha_k\tau}-1) + \tau\{j(e^{\alpha_k\tau}-1) - e^{\alpha_k\tau}\} \right] A_k$.

Calculating the inverse (I^{-1}) of I, determined by Eqs. 12-14, the asymptotic variances of the parameters (α_i's and A_i's) are obtained as the diagonal elements.

Section 2 of the previous chapter considers situations in which the observation is independent of the sampling interval and the count expectation is given by

$$\langle n_j \rangle = \sum A_j e^{-\alpha_i \tau}.$$

In this situation, the (k, l) elements of I become simpler and are calculated as follows:

$$I_{kl}^{(1,1)} = \sum_{j=1}^{m} \left\{ \frac{1}{\langle n_j \rangle} A_k A_l e^{-(\alpha_k+\alpha_l)(j-1)\tau} \times (j-1)^2 \tau^2 \right\}, \tag{15}$$

$$I_{kl}^{(2,2)} = \sum_{j=1}^{m} \left\{ \frac{1}{\langle n_j \rangle} e^{-(\alpha_k+\alpha_l)(j-1)\tau} \right\}, \tag{16}$$

$$I_{kl}^{(1,2)} = \sum_{j=1}^{m} \left\{ \frac{-1}{\langle n_j \rangle} A_k e^{-(\alpha_k+\alpha_l)(j-1)\tau} \times (j-1)\tau \right\}, \tag{17}$$

where $t_j = (j-1)\tau$ $(j=1, 2, \cdots, m)$ in this case.

2.2 EVALUATION OF ASYMPTOTIC VARIANCE IN NUMERICAL EXPERIMENTS

(1) Effect of sample size and sampling interval on asymptotic variance

Consider the dynamics of a 2-compartment system, i.e., a test function with two exponential terms

$$A_1 e^{-\alpha_1 t} + A_2 e^{-\alpha_2 t} = 20 e^{-0.05t} + 50 e^{-0.2t}.$$

The asymptotic variances of the parameters A_1, A_2, α_1 and α_2 were calculated for the different sample sizes 50, 100, 200, 500 and 1,000. The sampling intervals were also varied at values between 0.1 and 10. The relation between the variances and the sampling intervals ($V-\tau$ curves) is displayed on logarithmic scales (Fig. 1). Curves that are convex downward were obtained for each parameter and show that an optimal sampling interval exists, which minimizes the asymptotic variance. Bergner et al.[1] have shown an optimal sampling interval does exist.

The reason it does is that a decrease in the sampling interval when the sample size remains constant implies that only the initial slope of the dynamic curve is utilized; an increase in the sampling interval implies that the local features of the curve are overlooked. In either case the variance is increased.

Then, using the same test function, the sample size was increased with the sampling interval being kept constant ($\tau=1$). The asymptotic variance decreased significantly for sample size up to 100 and approached a constant value with continued increase in the sample size (Fig. 2). In other words, when the sampling interval is already specified, an increase in sample size beyond a certain level does not decrease the variance.

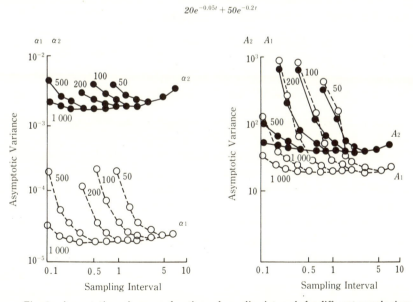

$$20e^{-0.05t} + 50e^{-0.2t}$$

Fig. 1. Asymptotic variances as functions of sampling intervals for different sample sizes.

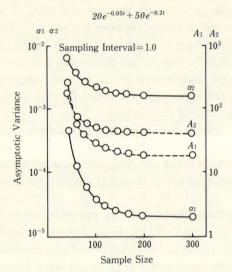

Fig. 2. Asymptotic variances as functions of sample size for fixed sampling interval ($\tau=1$).

(2) Effect of number of exponential terms on asymptotic variance

The V-τ relationship when the number of exponential terms is varied, was examined using the following functions:

(a) $q_1(t)=A_1 e^{-\alpha_1 t}=20e^{-0.05t}$.

(b) $q_2(t)=\sum_{i=1}^{2} A_i e^{-\alpha_i t}=20e^{-0.05t}+50e^{-0.2t}$.

(c) $q_3(t)=\sum_{i=1}^{3} A_i e^{-\alpha_i t}=20e^{-0.05t}+50e^{-0.2t}+30e^{-0.1t}$.

(d) $q_4(t)=\sum_{i=1}^{4} A_i e^{-\alpha_i t}=20e^{-0.05t}+50e^{-0.2t}+30e^{-0.1t}+5e^{-0.01t}$.

The asymptotic variances were calculated for $m=100$. For convenience in comparing the parameter variances, the test function with the larger number of exponential terms was constructed to include the function with a smaller number of exponential terms. Asymptotic variance can be seen to increase with the exponential terms, a tendency that is more pronounced for $q_4(t)$, which has the largest number of exponential terms (Fig. 3).

The slope of the V-τ curve is steeper near the minimum variance (V_{min}) when the number of exponential terms increases to 3 or 4. On the other hand, the V-τ curve for functions with 1 or 2 exponentials varies less near the V_{min}. Consequently, the sampling interval should be determined

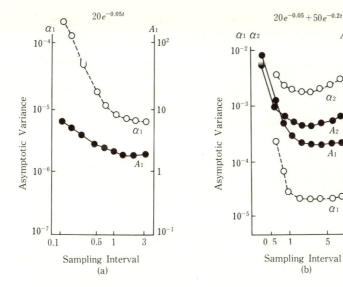
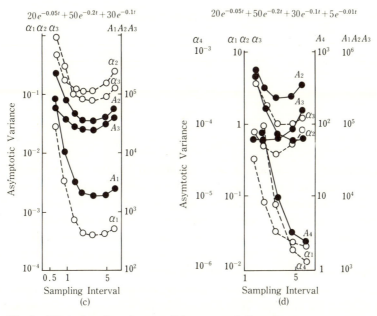

Fig. 3. Effect of number of exponentials on asymptotic variances.

solely in the parameter estimation for functions with more than 3 exponential terms.

The sampling interval corresponding to V_{min} shifts to the right (i.e., increases) with an increase in the number of exponential terms. When the function has a pair of similar exponents, asymptotic variances are generally larger for parameters of exponential terms close to each other.

(3) Optimal sampling interval

Now consider the sum of asymptotic variances normalized by squaring the values for parameters:

$$\sum \frac{\hat{\sigma}_i^2}{\theta_i^2} = \sum \left[E\left\{ \left(\frac{\hat{\theta}_i}{\theta_i} - 1 \right)^2 \right\} \right],$$

where $\hat{\sigma}_i^2$ is the asymptotic variance of θ_i corresponding to the ith diagonal element of I^{-1} (the inverse of Fisher's information matrix).

Here again the test functions used in section 2 of the previous chapter are noted. The asymptotic variances were calculated using Eqs. 15-17. Table 1 shows the optimal sampling intervals for $y_1(t)$, $y_2(t)$, and $y_3(t)$ computed for the three sample sizes.

Table 1. The optimal sampling intervals for $y_1(t)$, $y_2(t)$ and $y_3(t)$ at sample sizes 50, 100 and 200

Test function	Sample size		
	50	100	200
$Y_1(t)$	6.0	3.0	1.5
$Y_2(t)$	8.0	4.0	2.0
$Y_3(t)$	5.0	2.5	1.2

Parameters A_i, α_i and p were estimated for the optimal sampling interval, using the method described in the previous chapter. No substantial improvement was obtained for $y_1(t)$ and $y_2(t)$ because accurate identification had already been achieved without using these optimal sampling intervals. As for $y_3(t)$, recall that p was underestimated with $m=50$ and $\tau=1$. As shown in Table 2, p for $y_3(t)$ was successfully estimated, even with $m=50$, when the optimal sampling interval $\tau=5$ was used.

The accuracy of estimates of A_1 and α_1 was also improved by using the optimal sampling interval. However, results for $y_3(t)$ with $m=50$ were still unsatisfactory due to large asymptotic variances; values were 0.14×

Table 2. Estimation of parameters A_i, α_i and p for $y_3(t)$ at sample size 50, 100, and 200 with optimal sampling intervals

$$Y_3(t) = 100e^{-0.02t} + 200e^{-0.05t} + 300e^{-0.2t}$$

Sample size (m) & Sampling interval (τ)	1	2	Order 3 (1/2 AIC value)	4	Estimation of each parameter
m=50, τ=5.0	438.2	165.6	<u>159.8</u>	166.8	$71e^{-0.007t} + 197e^{-0.036t} + 346e^{-0.188t}$
m=100, τ=2.5	772.1	325.8	<u>317.7</u>	319.7	$106e^{-0.01t} + 232e^{-0.055t} + 291e^{-0.235t}$
m=200, τ=1.2	1439.8	643.2	<u>629.4</u>	638.8	$108e^{-0.01t} + 224e^{-0.055t} + 291e^{-0.203t}$

10^{-5}, 0.38×10^{-3}, 0.52×10^{-2}, 418, 7151, and 9456 for α_1, α_2, α_3, A_1, A_2, and A_3, respectively.

These data suggest that the sample size should be increased when asymptotic variances are still large, even when the optimal sampling intervals are used.

2.3 CONCLUDING REMARKS

The observation from the compartmental system is represented by a sum of exponential functions with Poisson fluctuation. Asymptotic variances of parameters in the maximum likelihood estimation were calculated using Fisher's information matrix and Cramer-Rao's inequality. From numerical experiments, the following conclusions were drawn.

1. Each sample size has an optimal sampling interval that minimizes the asymptotic variances of A_i and α_i.
2. With an increase in sample size but a constant sampling interval, asymptotic variance decreases, converging to a certain value.
3. With an increase in the number of exponential terms, the parameter variance is increased. This tendency is more pronounced for a system that includes four or more compartments.
4. The optimal sampling interval yields more accurate results in estimates of α_i, A_i, and p.

3. ASYMPTOTIC VARIANCE OF PARAMETER ESTIMATION IN THE COMPARTMENTAL SYSTEM WITH KNOWN STRUCTURE[6]

As mentioned, the linear compartmental system is represented by

$$\frac{d}{dt}x(t) = Ax(t) + b(t), \tag{18}$$

where $x'=(x_1, \cdots, x_p)$ denotes the state, $b'=(b_1, \cdots, b_p)$ the input, and $A \equiv \{a_{ij}\}$ the rate constant. The problem is to estimate the rate constants among compartments from the observed dynamic response of the input tracer.

Section 2 of this chapter considered the special case in which the mean value function of the output equals the sum of exponential functions. In this section the method used to calculate the asymptotic variance of the rate constant a_{ij} is given in Eq. 18, i.e., the asymptotic variance of parameters when the structure of the compartmental system is given beforehand. This situation is the same as that in section 3 of the previous chapter.

3.1 METHODS

Assume that $r \times m$ independent observations are made in compartments $1, 2, \cdots, r$ at times $t_1, t_2, \cdots, t_m$ and the observed vector at t_j is given by

$$n(t_j) \equiv \{n_1(t_j), n_2(t_j), \cdots, n_r(t_j)\}, \quad j=1, 2, \cdots, m. \tag{19}$$

The RI count at t_j is the time integral of the state x_i between t_{j-1} and t_j, and the expected value of $n_i(t_j)$ is written as

$$\langle n_i(t_j) \rangle = \int_{t_{j-1}}^{t_j} x_i(t) dt, \quad i=1, 2, \cdots, r. \tag{20}$$

Since RI data obey a Poisson distribution, the likelihood function is given by

$$L = \prod_{k=1}^{r} \prod_{j=1}^{m} \frac{e^{-\langle n_k(t_j) \rangle} \cdot \langle n_k(t_j) \rangle^{n_k(t_j)}}{n_k(t_j)!}. \tag{21}$$

As discussed in section 2, the (l, m) element I_{lm} of Fisher's information matrix[3] I is written as

$$I_{lm} = \sum_{k,j} \frac{1}{\langle n_k(t_j) \rangle} \frac{\partial \langle n_k(t_j) \rangle}{\partial \theta_l} \frac{\partial \langle n_k(t_j) \rangle}{\partial \theta_m}, \tag{22}$$

where $\{\theta\}$ is the parameter corresponding to $\{a_{ij}\}$.

To calculate $\langle n_k(t_j) \rangle$ and $\partial \langle n_k(t_j) \rangle / \partial \theta_l$ in Eq. 22, differential equations with respect to these quantities are derived as follows: Integrating Eq. 18 from t_{j-1} to t_j and multiplying by A^{-1}, it follows that

$$\langle n(t_j) \rangle = A^{-1}\{x(t_j) - x(t_{j-1})\} - A^{-1} \int_{t_{j-1}}^{t_j} b(t) dt. \tag{23}$$

Differentiating Eq. 23 with respect to a_{pq} results in

$$\frac{\partial <n(t_j)>}{\partial a_{pq}} = \frac{\partial A^{-1}}{\partial a_{pq}}\left\{x(t_j)-x(t_{j-1})-\int_{t_{j-1}}^{t_j} b(t)dt\right\}$$
$$+ A^{-1}\left\{\frac{\partial x(t_j)}{\partial a_{pq}} - \frac{\partial x(t_{j-1})}{\partial a_{pq}}\right\}. \tag{24}$$

Differentiating $AA^{-1}=E$ (unit matrix), components of $\partial A^{-1}/\partial a_{pq}$ are obtained as follows:

$$\left.\begin{array}{l}\dfrac{\partial a_{il}^{-1}}{\partial a_{pq}} = a_{ql}^{-1}(a_{iq}^{-1}-a_{ip}^{-1}) \quad \text{for } p \neq q \\[2mm] \dfrac{\partial a_{il}^{-1}}{\partial a_{qq}} = -a_{iq}^{-1}a_{ql}^{-1} \quad \text{for } p=q\end{array}\right\}. \tag{25}$$

To calculate Eq. 24, another partial derivative, $\partial x/\partial a_{pq}$ must be obtained. Partial differentiation of Eq. 18 with respect to a_{pq} yields:

$$\frac{d}{dt}\left(\frac{\partial x}{\partial a_{pq}}\right) = \frac{\partial A}{\partial a_{pq}}x + A\frac{\partial x}{\partial a_{pq}}. \tag{26}$$

Hence, the partial derivative $\partial x/\partial a_{pq}$ in Eq. 24 can be calculated by solving Eq. 26 under the initial condition $(\partial x/\partial a_{pq})_{t=-0}=0$.

Thus, the procedure for estimating asymptotic variance is as follows: Step 1: give the structure of compartments, the values of rate constants a_{ij}, the position of input and output, and the input functions. Step 2: solve the simultaneous differential equations 18 and 26 for x and $\partial x/\partial a_{pq}$, respectively, and calculate $\partial A^{-1}/\partial a_{pq}$, using Eq. 25. Step 3: calculate $<n(t_j)>$ and $\partial <n(t_j)>/\partial a_{pq}$, $j=1, 2, \cdots, m$ by substituting the results of Step 2 into Eqs. 23 and 24, respectively. Step 4: calculate Fisher's information matrix by substituting the results of step 3 into Eq. 5. Step 5: take the inverse of Eq. 5. The diagonal elements of I^{-1} give the asymptotic variances of rate constants a_{ij}.

3.2 RESULTS AND CONCLUDING REMARKS

The models used in this section are the same as those in section 3 of the previous chapter, i.e., the two-compartment catenary system and the three-compartment cyclical system. Values for the rate constants are: $a_{21}=0.1$, $a_{12}=0.05$, $a_{01}=0.1$ and $b=500$ in model A, and $a_{21}=0.08$, $a_{32}=0.03$, $a_{13}=0.1$, $a_{01}=0.02$ and $b=800$ in model B. These are also the same as those given in the previous chapter.

The asymptotic variances $\hat{\sigma}$ were calculated by varying the sampling

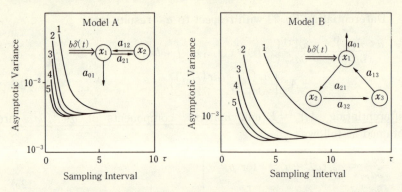

Fig. 4. Relationship between asymptotic variance and sampling interval. Variances for a_{01}, both in model A and B, are shown as representative cases. Figures 1, 2, ⋯, and 5 correspond to $m=20, 40, 60, 80,$ and 100, respectively.

interval with a fixed sample size, $m=50$. The results were given in Figure 3 of the preceding chapter. The vertical lines in that figure are estimates of parameters, including $\hat{\sigma}$; the horizontal lines are sampling intervals. Recall that downward convex curves were obtained for all "mean$+2\hat{\sigma}$" curves. These curves indicate that for each parameter, there is an optimal sampling interval that minimizes the asymptotic variance.

Asymptotic variances are then calculated for five different sample sizes. Figure 4 shows the asymptotic variances for a_{01} in models A and B. In general, an increase in sample size leads to a decrease in the optimal sampling interval τ_{opt} and also to a decrease in asymptotic variances corresponding to τ_{opt}.

In conclusion, the following were found:

1. There is also an optimal sampling interval that minimizes asymptotic variances of a_{ij} for each sample size.

2. Asymptotic variances provides a good measure of the accuracy of estimates of parameters in the compartmental system.

REFERENCES

1. Bergner, P.E., Takeuchi, K. & Lui, Y.Y.: The recognition problem: Application to sum of exponentials. *Math. Biosci.* 17: 315-337, 1973.
2. Wagner, H.N., Jr., Walton, W.W., Jr. & Jacquez, J.: Mathematics. In *Principles of Nuclear Medicine,* ed. H.N. Wagner, Jr., W.B. Saunders Co., Philadelphia, London, Toronto, 1968.
3. Fisher, R.A.: *Statistical Methods and Scientific Inference.* Hafner Press, New York, 1973.
4. Rao, C.R.: *Linear Statistical Inference and its Applications.* John Wiley & Sons, Inc., New York, 1965.
5. Kajiya, F., Kawagoe, K., Kodama, S. et al.: Optimum Sampling for Identification of Compartmental Systems. *Elect. & Comm. Japan* 59C, 69-76, Scripta Publ. Co., New York, 1976.
6. Kagiyama, M., Kajiya, F., Hoki, N. et al.: On an optimal sampling condition in the identification of compartmental system with known structure. *Trans. IECE Japan* E63: 865-866, 1980.

3
STRUCTURAL IDENTIFIABILITY OF LINEAR COMPARTMENTAL SYSTEMS

Hideo Kusuoka, Hajime Maeda and Shinzo Kodama

1. INTRODUCTION

This chapter considers the structural identifiability of compartmental systems. This concept, first posed by Bellman and Åström[1], is related to the following problem of parameter identification: Given both an input-output observation and *a priori* knowledge of the structure of connections among compartments, can unknown parameters (rate constants) be uniquely determined?

A precise definition of parameter identifiability, given by Glover and Willems, in terms of transfer functions maintains that no two distinct neighboring sets of parameters can have the same transfer function[2]. In other words, this definition requires that the map $F(\cdot)$ from the system parameters into the coefficients of the transfer function is locally injective (one-to-one). Many attempts have been made to obtain necessary and/or sufficient conditions to guarantee this one-to-one correspondence. However, a complete solution is not available at the present time. Delforge recently reported a new algorithm by which the structural identifiability of a given compartment system can be checked in terms of its graphic structure[3]. However, his proof contains some technical difficulties, as pointed out by Norton and others[4].

In this chapter, a new definition of structural identifiability is proposed. In practice, exact input-output data cannot be obtained: all that can be expected are data with random errors. We would like to determine approximate system parameters from such data. These should be close to the true parameters. Consequently, the map $F(\cdot)$ must be one-to-one and onto (surjective), and $F^{-1}(\cdot)$ must be continuous; the map $F(\cdot)$ is a homeomorphism. This requirement has been adopted as the definition of structural identifiability and provides the necessary and sufficient conditions for structural identifiability in terms of the Jacobian matrix $\partial F/\partial p$. Based on these results, several necessary conditions are then assigned to the structure of connections among the compartments, including input and output positions. By numerical assessment, using computers, these conditions are shown to be sufficient for 3- and 4-compartment systems; then the structural identifiability of these systems is characterized by the structure of their compartment interconnections, including input and output positions. The relationship of structural identifiability to closed and open systems as well as dual systems is discussed.

2. THE PROBLEM OF STRUCTURAL IDENTIFIABILITY

Consider linear time-invariant compartmental systems in the form of a state equation:

$$\dot{x} = Ax + bu,$$
$$y = c^T x, \qquad (1)$$

where A is an $n \times n$ real matrix, b and c are $n \times 1$ real vectors, and n is the number of compartments.

As is well known, the elements of matrix A are related to the rate constants of the system k_{ij}, by

$$\begin{aligned} a_{ij} &= k_{ij}, & (i \neq j,\ i, j = 1, 2, \cdots, n) \\ a_{ii} &= -k_{0i} - \sum_{j \neq i} k_{ji}. & (i = 1, 2, \cdots, n) \end{aligned} \qquad (2)$$

If all excretions are zero, i.e., $k_{0i} = 0$ for all i's, the system is said to be closed; otherwise it is an open system.

We then assume that the compartmental system has a set of fixed zero rate constants $k_{ij} = 0$, and the remaining rate constants take on arbitrary positive real values unrelated to each other.

Suppose an input is applied to one of the compartments, say the ith compartment, and its quantity in a certain compartment, say the jth compartment, is observed. Then we have

$$b = e_i\ (i\text{th unit vector}), \quad c = e_j\ (j\text{th unit vector}). \qquad (3)$$

The zero-state input-output relationship of Eq. 1 is completely characterized by the transfer function:

$$h(s) = e_j^T(sI-A)^{-1}e_i$$
$$= \frac{\delta_{ij}s^{n-1} + b_{n-2}s^{n-2} + \cdots + b_0}{s^n + a_{n-1}s^{n-1} + \cdots + a_1 s + a_0}, \qquad (4)$$

where $\delta_{ij} = 1 \quad (i=j)$
$\phantom{\text{where }\delta_{ij}} = 0 \quad (i \neq j).$

We note that the number of variable parameters a_i's and b_j's of the transfer function is given by:

$r = 2n-1 \quad$ (for open systems)
$ = 2n-2 \quad$ (for closed systems). $\qquad (5)$

To determine the unknown rate coefficients from the given transfer function with the help of Eq. 4, we introduce a map $F(\cdot)$ from the unknown rate constants to the r-variable coefficients of the transfer function:

$$z = F(p), \qquad (6)$$

where $p = \text{col}[p_1, p_2, \cdots, p_q]$ is the vector consisting of the unknown rate constants, and z is the vector of the variable coefficients of the transfer function, i.e.,

$z = \text{col}[a_0, a_1, \cdots, a_{n-1}, b_0, b_1, \cdots, b_{n-2}], (r=2n-1)$ for open systems
$ = \text{col}[a_1, a_2, \cdots, a_{n-1}, b_0, b_1, \cdots, b_{n-2}], (r=2n-2)$ for closed systems.
$\qquad (7)$

Much of the literature focuses attention on the one-to-one correspondence of the map $F(\cdot)$, and hence it is assumed that $q \leq r$.

If $q < r$, then the problem of solving Eq. 6 is ill-posed and numerical difficulties occur[5]. Therefore, in the following, we assume that $q = r$, i.e., the number of unknown parameters is equal to $2n-1$ ($2n-2$) for open (closed) systems. Moreover, we would like the unique solution p of Eq. 6 to depend continuously on a given vector z, to ensure that small observational errors are responsible for the error between the approximate and true solutions. Thus, structural identifiability is defined as follows:

Definition 1: A compartmental system is said to be structurally identifiable if $r = q$ and the map $F(\cdot)$, given by Eq. 6, is a local homeomorphism almost everywhere in p.

Remark: The term "almost everywhere" implies that a property Π may fail only on a closed proper subset $V = \{p | \Psi(p_1, p_2, \cdots, P_q) = 0\}$, where Ψ is a polynomial; in other words, it holds for an open dense subset[6].

Structural Identifiability of Linear Compartmental Systems

The following theorem can be derived from Definition 1. This theorem plays a fundamental role in this discussion.

Theorem 1: Map F, defined in Eq. 6, is a local homeomorphism for almost every p if and only if $\det[\partial F/\partial p] \neq 0$ for almost every p.

Remark: As pointed out in Reference 2, Definition 1 is equivalent to requiring that the map $G(\cdot)$, from the unknown rate constants to the Markov parameters $\{c^T A^k b\}_{k=1}^r$, is a local homeomorphism almost everywhere.

$G(\cdot)$ can be read directly from the flow graph associated with the compartment matrix A in which a node corresponds to the individual compartment, and if $a_{ji} \neq 0$ there is an edge from node i to node j with associated weight a_{ji}. The flow graph has self loops of weight a_{ii} ($i=1, 2, \cdots, n$). Let w be the vector consisting of a_{ii}, then, $G(\cdot)$ is given as

$$z = G(p) = f(p, g(p))$$

or

$$z = f(p, w),$$
$$w = g(p), \qquad (8)$$

where $f(\cdot, \cdot)$ denotes the relation between Markov parameters $c^T A^k b$ ($k=1, 2, \cdots, r$) and p, w; and $g(\cdot)$ the relation between a_{ii} and p_i (see Eq. 2).

3. NECESSARY CONDITIONS FOR STRUCTURAL IDENTIFIABILITY

In this section, several necessary conditions for structural identifiability are given in terms of the structure of connections among compartments. As a sequel, a compartmental system is a driving point (DP) system, if input and output positions are the same; otherwise it is a transfer (T) system. Throughout this chapter, the number of unknown rate constants is assumed to be $2n-1(2n-2)$ for open (closed) systems, and an open system has exactly one excretion.

The following terms are defined to describe the theorems:

Sufficiently connectedness: A compartmental system is said to be *sufficiently connected* if there is a Menger-type complete linking in the representation graph of Eq. 8. Here the graph is a directed graph in which the node set is $\{z_1, \cdots, z_r\}$, $\{w_1, \cdots, w_n\}$, $\{p_1, \cdots, p_n\}$, and if the expression $z_i = f_i(p, w)$ contains p_j and w_j, then there are edges from node p_j and node w_j to node z_i; if the expression $w_k=g_k(p)$ contains p_l, then there is an edge from node p_l to node w_k. Menger-type linking means the set of disjoint directed paths from $\{p\}$ to $\{z\}$, and if the number of such directed paths is equal to r, the number of $\{z_k\}$, then the linking is said to be complete.

Remark: We can show that for sufficiently connectedness, it is necessary that in the set of Markov parameters $c^T A^k b (k=1, 2, \cdots, r)$, no subset exists that contains strictly less than m distinct unknown rate constants p_1, $p_2, \cdots, p_{m-k}$ ($1 \le k \le m-1$). Here parameters p_j's are not counted as distinct entities if the p_i's are included in the subset in the form of a sum, Σp_i.

It is known that if $\partial f_i / \partial p_j$, $\partial f_i / \partial w_j$ and $\partial g_i / \partial p_j$ are independent, then $\det[\partial G / \partial p] \ne 0$ if and only if there is a Menger-type complete linking in the representation graph of Eq. 8[10]. Hence, it can be concluded that the system is structurally identifiable if and only if it is sufficiently connected in the above sense. However, in our problem we can *not* expect partial derivatives to be independent.

Source, sink and transit: The digraph of a compartmental system can be decomposed into a collection of strongly connected subgraphs[7]; each subgraph falls into one of the following categories:
1. *Source*: Strongly connected subgraph with no couplings directed toward any of its compartments.
2. *Sink*: Strongly connected subgraph with no couplings directed away from any of its compartments.
3. *Transit*: Strongly connected subgraph with at least one coupling directed away from one of its compartments, and at least one coupling directed toward one of its compartments.

Receiving compartment: The receiving compartment is just a single compartment that receives all couplings toward the sink from other digraphs (Fig. 1). If the sink consists of a single compartment, then by definition it is the receiving compartment.

Using these terms, the necessary conditions for structural identifiability are as follows[8].

Theorem 2: A DP compartmental system is structurally identifiable only if the following conditions are satisfied: (a) the system is sufficiently connected and (b) it does not contain an unidentifiable subsystem (see Fig. 2).

Theorem 3: A closed, T-compartmental system is structurally identifiable only if the following conditions are satisfied: (a) the system is sufficiently connected, (b) it does not contain an unidentifiable subsys-

Structural Identifiability of Linear Compartmental Systems 41

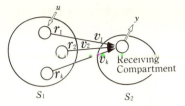

Fig. 1. Definition of the receiving compartment.

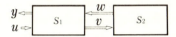

Fig. 2. If subsystem S_2 is not structurally identifiable, the overall system is not structurally identifiable.

tem, and (c) there is no sink containing the receiving compartment.

Theorem 4: An open, T-compartmental system is structurally identifiable only if the following conditions are satisfied: (a) the system is sufficiently connected, (b) it does not contain an unidentifiable subsystem, (c) there is no sink containing the receiving compartment, and (d) if a sink exists, the excretion is restricted to the sink.

4. NECESSARY AND SUFFICIENT CONDITION FOR 3- AND 4-COMPARTMENT SYSTEMS

In this section, we consider 3- and 4-compartment systems and show that the necessary conditions stated in the previous section are also sufficient for these systems. To determine whether or not the system is structurally identifiable, the nonsingularity of $\partial G/\partial p$ must be checked. This is accomplished numerically by the Monte Carlo method.

The following result is useful to exclude substantial numbers of systems when the nonsingularity of $\partial G/\partial p$ is examined.

Lemma: The following is a set of necessary conditions for sufficiently connectedness.

DP system: (a) compartment diagram is strongly connected, and (b) at least one compartment has edges both toward and away from the I/O compartment.

T system: (a) The number of source subgraphs is, at most, one, and the number of sink subgraphs is also, at most, one. The input is applied to the source, and output is observed at the sink. (b) There is a direct edge from input to output.

4.1 DP-SYSTEM

By exhaustive numerical assessment by computer with all possible compartmental systems satisfying the conditions of the Lemma, we have found that in this class of systems the 3rd order DP systems are all structurally identifiable; and the 4th order DP systems are structurally identifiable except for the systems shown in Figure 3. Note that each of the systems in Figure 3 has an unidentifiable subsystem of order 2. Thus, we conclude that the conditions of Theorem 2 are necessary and sufficient for 3- and 4-compartment systems to be structurally identifiable.

4.2 T-SYSTEM

As in the case of DP-systems, we apply a numerical assessment to all possible compartmental structures satisfying the conditions of Lemma. The computer experiment shows that the 3rd order unidentifiable systems are either those with receiving compartments or the one shown in Figure 4. The system of Figure 4 has an excretion from the source, which violates condition (d) of Theorem 4. Thus, we conclude that the conditions of Theorems 3 and 4 are necessary and sufficient for the structural identifiability of 3-compartment T-systems.

The fourth order unidentifiable systems are listed in Table 1. Each row in Table 1 denotes the structure generated from the seven standard structures given in Figure 5: "1" ("0") means that the corresponding edge has the same (reverse) direction and IN (OUT) denotes the input (output) position. "x" implies that the system is unidentifiable. Because of space limitations, among the unidentifiable systems generated from Type I, only systems that satisfy the conditions of the Lemma as well as condition (c)

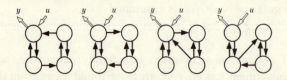

Fig. 3. Unidentifiable structures of 4-compartment DP systems.

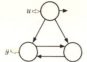

Fig. 4. Unidentifiable structure of 3-compartment T-systems.

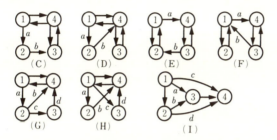

Fig. 5. Standard structures of 4-compartment systems.

of Theorem 3 and Theorem 4 are listed. Note that each of the systems in Table 1 violates at least one of the conditions (b) to (d) of Theorem 3 and Theorem 4. Thus, we conclude that the conditions of Theorem 3 and Theorem 4 are necessary and sufficient for the structural identifiability of 4-compartment T-systems.

5. RELATIONS BETWEEN CLOSED AND OPEN SYSTEMS AND THE DUALITY IN STRUCTURAL IDENTIFIABILITY

In this section, the relationship between closed and open systems as well as that among dual systems, with regard to structural identifiability, are considered. A dual system is defined as follows: given a compartmental system S, we construct its dual S_d as the system in which (a) all edges except leakages are reversed, and (b) the input (output) compartment of S is the output (input) compartment of S_d. The following theorems are then proved[9]:

Theorem 5: If a DP compartmental system is structurally identifiable, then the dual DP system is also structurally identifiable.

Theorem 6: Consider an open DP system with only one excretion and the corresponding closed DP system obtained by neglecting the excretion.

Table 1. List of unidentifiable structures of 4th order T and DP compartmental systems (See the text)

	Direction				IN	OUT	closed	Excretion			
	a	b	c	d				1	2	3	4
C-1	1	0	1	1	1	2	X	X	X	X	X
C-2	0	1	1	1	2	1		X	X		
D-1	1	0	1	1	1	2	X	X	X		
D-2	1	0	1	0	4	2	X	X	X	X	X
D-3	0	0	1	1	2	1			X	X	
D-4	0	1	1	1	2	4		X	X		
E-1	1	1	1	1	1	2	X	X	X	X	X
E-2	1	1	0	1	2	1	X	X	X	X	
E-3	1	0	0	1	1	4			X	X	
F-1	1	1	1	1	1	2	X	X	X	X	X
F-2	1	1	0	1	2	1	X	X	X	X	X
F-3	1	0	1	0	1	4		X	X	X	X
F-4	0	1	0	1	4	1	X	X	X	X	
G-1	1	1	1	1	2	3	X	X	X	X	X
G-2	1	0	1	1	2	3	X	X	X	X	X
G-3	1	0	1	0	4	2	X	X	X	X	X
G-4	1	1	0	0	3	2	X	X	X	X	X
G-5	0	0	0	0	1	2	X	X	X	X	X
G-6	1	0	0	0	3	2	X		X	X	X
G-7	1	0	0	1	4	2	X	X			
G-8	0	1	1	1	2	1		X	X	X	
G-9	0	1	1	1	2	3			X	X	X
G-10	0	0	1	1	2	4			X	X	X
G-11	0	0	0	0	3	2	X		X	X	X
G-12	1	1	0	0	3	2	X	X	X	X	
G-13	1	1	1	0	2	3	X	X	X	X	
G-14	1	1	1	0	4	3	X	X	X	X	X
G-15	0	1	1	0	2	3	X	X	X	X	
G-16	1	0	1	0	4	3	X	X	X	X	
G-17	0	0	1	0	4	3	X	X	X	X	
G-18	0	0	1	0	2	3			X	X	
G-19	1	1	0	1	3	4				X	
G-20	1	1	0	1	3	2			X	X	
G-21	0	1	0	1	3	4			X	X	
G-22	1	0	0	1	3	2	X		X	X	X
G-23	0	0	0	1	3	4				X	
G-24	0	0	0	1	3	2					
H-1	1	0	1	1	1	2		X	X	X	
H-2	1	1	0	1	4	2	X	X	X	X	
H-3	0	1	1	1	2	1			X		
H-4	0	1	1	1	2	4				X	
I-1	0	0	0	0	1	2		X	X	X	X
I-2	0	0	0	1	1	2	X	X	X	X	X
I-3	0	1	1	1	1	2	X	X	X	X	X
I-4	1	0	1	0	1	2	X	X	X	X	X
I-5	0	1	1	1	1	2	X	X	X	X	X
I-6	0	1	1	0	1	2	X	X	X	X	X
I-7	0	1	0	0	1	2	X	X	X	X	X
I-8	1	1	0	0	1	2	X	X	X	X	X
I-9	0	1	0	1	1	2	X	X	X	X	X
I-10	1	0	1	1	1	2	X	X	X	X	X
I-11	1	1	1	1	1	2	X	X	X	X	X

If one is structurally identifiable, then the other is also structurally identifiable.

Theorem 7 : Consider T-compartmental systems. If a closed system is structurally identifiable, the open system with only one excretion is structurally identifiable.

Remark : In T-compartmental system, the structural identifiability is not necessarily shared among dual systems. Also, it should be noted that the structural identifiability of an open system does not always imply that of the closed system.

6. CONCLUSION

In this chapter, the problem of the structural identifiability of linear time-invariant compartmental systems has been investigated. A necessary and sufficient condition for structural identifiability has been given in terms of the Jacobian matrix of the map, from unknown rate constants to variable coefficients of the transfer function. Based on these results, several necessary conditions have been derived in terms of the structures of connections among compartments. By numerical assessment using computers, it has been shown that for 3- and 4-compartment systems, these conditions are also sufficient.

The two problems concerning the relationship between open and closed systems and the duality of systems are discussed from the viewpoint of structural identifiability.

REFERENCES

1. Bellman, R. & Åström, K.J : On structural identifiability. *Math. Biosci.* 7 : 329-339, 1970.
2. Glover, K. & Willems, J.C. : Parametrization of linear dynamical systems : Canonical forms and identifiability. *IEEE Trans.* AC-19 : 640-645, 1974.
3. Delforge, J. : Necessary and sufficient structural condition for local identifiability of a system with linear compartments. *Math. Biosci.* 54 : 159-180, 1981.
4. Norton, J.P. : Letter to the Editor. *Math. Biosci.* 61 : 295-298, 1982.
5. Ortega, J.M. & Rheinbold, W.C. : *Iterative solution of nonlinear equation in several variables.* Academic Press, New York, 1970.
6. Wonham, W.H. : *Linear multivariable control, A geometric approach.* Springer-Verlag, New York, 1974.
7. Zazworsky, R.M. & Kundesen, H.K. : Structural controllability and observability of linear time-invariant compartmental models. *IEEE Trans.* AC-23 : 872-877, 1978.
8. Okano, S., Maeda, H., Kodama, S. et al. : A study on structural identifiability of compart-

mental systems. *Trans. IECE* J64-A : 203-210, 1981 (in Japanese).
9   Maeda, H., Okano, S., Kodama, S. et al.: A graphical aspect of structural identifiability of compartmental systems. *Trans. SICE* 17 : 455-460, 1981 (in Japanese).
10 Iri, M., Tsunekawa, J. & Murota, K.: Graph-theoretic approach to large-scale systems of equations-structured solvability and block-triangularization. *Trans. Inform. Proc. Soc. Japan* 23 : 88-95, 1982 (in Japanese).

1

REALIZATION PROBLEMS IN LINEAR COMPARTMENTAL SYSTEMS

Hajime Maeda and Shinzo Kodama

1. INTRODUCTION

This chapter considers problems related to the realization of linear time-invariant compartmental systems; the objective here is to give some results as well as to point out difficulties in the problem and thus gain a theoretical insight into the input-output properties of such systems.

By a linear time invariant compartmental system, we mean a system described by the state equation[1]

$$\dot{x} = Ax + bu, \quad y = c^T x, \tag{1}$$
$$A = [a_{ij}] \in R^{n \times n}, \quad b = [b_1, \cdots, b_n]^T \in R^n, \quad c = [c_1, \cdots, c_n]^T \in R^n,$$

where $x = [x_1, x_2, \cdots, x_n]^T$ is the state with x_i, $i = 1, 2, \cdots, n$, denoting the amount of material of interest in the ith compartment, u is the input and y is the output to be measured. The entries of A are related to the rate constants k_{ij} by $a_{ij} = k_{ij} (i \neq j)$ and $a_{ii} = -k_{0i} - \sum_{j \neq i} k_{ji}$, where k_{ij} is the rate constant for the flow from compartment j to i, and k_{0i} is the rate of excretion from compartment i. As the rate constants, as well as entries in b (input vector) and c (observation vector), are non-negative, the constraints that characterize a compartmental system are:

$$b_i \geq 0, \, c_i \geq 0, \quad i = 1, 2, \cdots, n \tag{2}$$
$$a_{ij} \geq 0, \quad i \neq j \tag{3}$$
$$a_{ii} \leq 0, \quad i = 1, 2, \cdots, n \tag{4}$$

It is known that with constraints (2)-(4), the dynamic behavior of compartmental system (1) exhibits certain characteristics (e.g., stability and non-negativity of solutions)[3]. In this chapter it will be shown that the constraints also cause difficulty in the realization problem.

Roughly speaking, realization is the process of building a model from given input-output (I/O) data. Here we mean that a realization problem is one in which a compartmental system must be found from a given system function. More specifically, the problem is: given a system function $H(s)$, find A, b, c satisfying Eqs. 2-4 such that $H(s) = c^T(sI - A)^{-1}b$.

A number of researchers have considered the realization problem[2-5]. At present, however, the complete solution is not known. Schoenfeld and Berman[2] first derived a necessary and sufficient condition for a system function $H(s)$ to be realized as the driving point function of a 3-compartment system; moreover, they obtained a *canonical* form 3-compartment realization. They also gave — with the aid of the electrical network theory — a necessary and sufficient condition for an $H(s)$ to be realized as the driving point function of a *catenary* or a *mammillary* system. Rubinow and Winzer[4] considered 2-, 3- and 4-compartment systems in detail and gave canonical-form compartmental systems, together with a procedure to determine the rate constants. In the following, we extend these results and, at the same time, point out a difficulty inherent in the problem.

In Section 2, realizability conditions are considered first. Realizability is equivalent to compatibility of I/O data with the compartmental representation. A system function $H(s)$ is *compartment-realizable* (or simply C-realizable) if it has representation (1), with (A, b, c) satisfying the constraints (2), (3) and (4). Observe that without the constraints, the realization problem is trivial, because it is known that a system function $H(s)$ is realized in the form (1) if, and only if, $H(s)$ is rational and proper[6]. In Section 2 we only consider a compartmental system in which the input is applied to a single compartment and the output is also observed through a single (not necessarily the same) compartment. First, some general observations are given and then a complete solution of the realizability for a system function of degree 3 or less is stated. This is a generalization of Schoenfeld and Berman in that (a) their consideration is limited to the *driving point* system functions, and (b) in their problem the number of compartments is *a priori* known. Second, we consider a class of compartmental systems having *non-cyclic* structures. This is a generalization of the mammillary and catenary systems. We give a necessary and sufficient condition for an nth order system function to be realized by a non-cyclic compartmental system.

In Section 3, we consider the dimension of realization, i.e., the number of compartments required for realization. Specifically, we consider the minimum possible dimension associated with realization. Again, this is a trivial problem if no constraints are placed on (A, b, c), because in this case the minimal dimension is equal to the McMillan degree of the system function, and a minimal realization (A, b, c) is both controllable and observable[6]. With regard to compartment-realization at hand, we cannot expect that the same properties hold. Indeed, an example is given to show that the minimal dimension is greater than the McMillan degree. This means that realization may require the introduction of uncontrollable and/or unobservable compartments to satisfy the required constraints.

2. REALIZABILITY CONDITION

Henceforth a real square matrix A that satisfies Eqs. 3 and 4 is called a compartment or C-matrix and is denoted by $A \in C$. In the following, it is assumed that the input is applied to a single compartment (say the kth compartment) and that the output is also observed at a single compartment (say the mth compartment). Hence, b and c are unit vectors e_k and e_m, respectively. A rational function $H(s)$ is said to be C-realizable if $A \in C$, e_k, e_m and positive number $\alpha > 0$ exist, such that

$$H(s) = \alpha \cdot e_m^T (sI - A)^{-1} e_k. \qquad (5)$$

The quadruplet (A, e_k, e_m, α) in Eq. 5 is said to be a realization of $H(s)$.

It is well known that $A \in C$ has no eigenvalues in the open right half plane and no purely imaginary ones; moreover zero eigenvalue, if it exists, is a simple root of the minimal polynomial of A[3]. It is also known that if $A \in C$, then the state transition matrix $\exp[At]$ is non-negative for all $t \geq 0$[3] (each element of $\exp[At]$ is non-negative for $t \geq 0$). From these facts and from Eq. 5, we can deduce the following general properties of system functions (i.e., necessary conditions for $H(s)$ to be C-realizable):

(P 1) $H(s)$ is stable in the sense that all poles are in the closed left half plane and the pole on the imaginary axis, if it exists, is at the origin with multiplicity 1.

(P 2) The inverse Laplace transform of $H(s)$ (i.e., impulse response) is non-negative for all $t \geq 0$.

As we shall see in the following, when restrictions are placed on the input and output positions, we obtain more useful necessary conditions.

2.1 REALIZABILITY OF DRIVING POINT FUNCTIONS

As for a driving point function, we may assume, without loss of generality, that the compartment for which the input is applied and the output is observed is compartment 1: thus, a driving point function (DPF) is assumed to be of the form

$$H(s) = e_1^T(sI - A)^{-1} e_1, \qquad (6)$$

where $e_1 = \text{col}[1, 0, \cdots, 0]$.

Theorem 1[5]: The driving point function $H(s)$ in Eq. 6 has the following properties:
1. $H(s)$ is a strictly proper *positive real* function.
2. Let $h(t)$ be the impulse response, i.e., $h(t) = e_1^T \exp[At] e_1$. Then, $h(0) \geq h(t) \geq 0$ for all $t \geq 0$.
3. $\dot{h}(0) < 0$.

This theorem shows that the realization problem is related to that of an electrical network. It is known that a rational function is realized as the driving point impedance function of a passive RLC-network if and only if it is positive real. This means that the set of C-realizable functions is a subclass of DPFs of passive RLC-networks. Moreover, it is known that the driving point impedance function of an RC-network $(Z_{RC})^*$ is always realizable as the DPF of compartmental system[2]. Thus, the class of C-realizable functions is larger than Z_{RC}.

Now we know that a system function $H(s)$ is C-realizable if it is a Z_{RC}-function. This can be extended as shown in Theorem 2 below.

Theorem 2[5]: Let $H(s)^{-1} = s + a - G(s)$, and suppose
(a) $a \geq G(0) \geq 0$.
(b) $G(s)$ is decomposable as

$$G(s) = \frac{c_1}{s + \sigma_{n-1}} + \cdots + \frac{c_{n-1}}{(s + \sigma_{n-1}) \cdots (s + \sigma_1)},$$

where $c_i \geq 0$, $\sigma_i > 0$ for $i = 1, 2, \cdots, n-1$.
Then $H(s)$ is realizable as a DPF of a compartmental system and, moreover, it has a realization with dimension n.

Note that any Z_{RC}-function can be decomposed to satisfy the conditions of Theorem 2.

* $H(s) \in Z_{RC}$ has simple poles and simple zeros on the non-positive real axis, and each zero separates the poles.

Now consider the case where the degree of $H(s) \leq 3$, and apply Theorem 2 to $H(s)$. Then in view of Theorem 1, the following is necessary and sufficient for $H(s)$ to be realizable as a DPF of a compartmental system.

$$H(s)^{-1} = s + a - [h_1/(s+\sigma_2) + h_2/(s+\sigma_1)(s+\sigma_2)] \qquad (7)$$
$$(h_1 \geq 0, h_2 \geq 0, \sigma_2 \geq \sigma_1 > 0, a \geq h_1\sigma_2^{-1} + h_2\sigma_1^{-1}\sigma_2^{-1})$$

Realizability condition Eq. 7 was first derived in 2 by examining the DPF of 3-compartment systems. Namely, Schoenfeld and Berman[2] have shown that Eq. 7 with $h_2 > 0$ is necessary and sufficient for $H(s)$ to be realized by the DPF of a 3-compartment system. Their result does not rule out the possibility that a DPF of degree 3 exists, which does *not* have a 3-compartment realization but which permits a *4 or higher* compartment realization. In this respect, the above assertion becomes somewhat stronger. It says that any realizable function of degree 3 is *always* realized by a 3-compartment system.

2.2 REALIZABILITY OF TRANSFER FUNCTIONS

To make a distinction from a DPF, in the following we specifically say that $H(s)$ is a transfer function (TF) of a compartmental system if

$$H(s) = a \cdot e_m^T(sI - A)^{-1} e_k, \ A \in C, \ a > 0, \ m \neq k. \qquad (8)$$

Note that the TF of compartmental systems is a strictly proper rational function in which the difference of degrees of numerator and denominator polynomials is greater than 2 and satisfies the general necessary conditions (P1) and (P2). As in the case of DPF, the general necessary and sufficient condition for realizability is not known. When the degree of $H(s) \leq 2$, then it is easy to see that a necessary and sufficient condition for $H(s)$ to be realized as a TF of compartmental systems is

$$H(s) = \frac{1}{(s+\sigma_1)(as+\sigma_2)} \quad (\sigma_2 \geq \sigma_1 \geq 0, \sigma_2 > 0, a \geq 0).$$

In this case, the minimal dimension is equal to the McMillan degree of $H(s)$.

2.3 TREE-COMPARTMENTAL SYSTEM REALIZATIONS

In 2.1 and 2.2, realizability as the problem of finding matrix $A \in C$ has

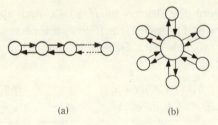

Fig. 1. Catenary system (a). Mammillary system (b).

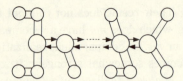

Fig. 2. Tree-compartmental system.

been considered. Here we consider the case in which compartmental system structure is *pre-assigned*, namely the graph of interconnections among compartments is given *a priori* (of course rate constants k_{ij} are still assumed to be non-negative and unknown).

Typical and useful compartmental structures are *catenary* and *mammillary* systems (see Fig. 1 (a) and (b)). A more general structure, including catenary and mammillary systems, is a tree structure. A *tree-compartmental system* is defined as follows: construct a non-oriented graph corresponding to the compartmental diagram so that a node denotes an individual compartment, and an edge between nodes i and j is drawn if at least one of k_{ij} and k_{ji} is not identically zero. If the non-oriented graph obtained by this procedure has no loop, then the system is called a tree-compartmental system (see Fig. 2). The matrix associated with a tree-compartmental (catenary, mammillary) system is referred to as a tree-compartmental (catenary, mammillary) matrix, and a function $H(s)$ is *tree (catenary, mammillary)-realizable* if a positive constant α, positive integers m and k, and a tree-compartmental (catenary, mammillary) matrix A exist such that

$$H(s) = \alpha \cdot e_m^T (sI - A)^{-1} e_k.$$

The properties of system functions of tree-compartmental systems are completely characterized by Z_{RC}-functions.

Theorem 3[5] : Necessary and sufficient conditions for $H(s)$ to be tree-realizable are : (a) the pole at the origin, if any, is simple and (b) $H(s)$ is a product of strictly proper Z_{RC}-functions $Z_i(s)(i=1, \cdots, r)$,

$$H(s)=Z_1(s)Z_2(s)\cdots Z_r(s).$$

Theorem 4[7] : Necessary and sufficient conditions for $H(s)$ to be catenary-realizable are : (a) the pole at the origin, if any, is simple and (b) $H(s)$ is a product of strictly proper Z_{RC}-functions $Z_i(s)(i=1, \cdots, r)$,

$$H(s)=Z_1(s)Z_2(s)\cdots Z_r(s),$$

where

$$Z_i(s)=\frac{1}{s+a_i} \quad (a_i>0) \text{ for } i=3, \cdots, r.$$

Theorem 5[8] : Necessary and sufficient conditions for $H(s)$ to be mammillary-realizable are : (a) the pole at the origin, if any, is simple; (b) $H(s)$ is a product of strictly proper Z_{RC}-functions $Z_i(s)$ $(i=1, \cdots, r)$

$$H(s)=Z_1(s)Z_2(s)\cdots Z_r(s),$$

where

$$Z_i(s)=\frac{1}{s+a_i} \quad (a_i>0) \text{ for } i=2, \cdots, r, \text{ and } r\leq 3$$

and (c) $H(s)$ has a pole with multiplicity 3 only if $H(s)$ is strictly stable, i.e., all poles are negative.

In Theorems 3 and 4, a realization is obtained by the *Cauer continued fraction expansion method*, and in Theorem 5 by the *Foster partial fraction expansion method*. In each case realization has the dimension equal to the McMillan degree of $H(s)$.

3. MINIMAL REALIZATIONS

In Section 2, we have shown several sufficient conditions for realizability, in which the minimal dimension is equal to the McMillan degree of the system function. As will be shown, this is not always the case, and all we can say is that, in general, minimal dimension is equal to or greater

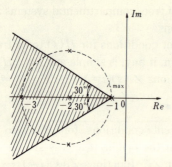

Fig. 3. Allowable eigenvalues location of 3×3 $A \in C$.

than the McMillan degree. That is, to obtain a minimal realization, we sometimes purposely introduce uncontrollable and/or unobservable parts to satisfy the constraints Eqs. 2-4.

Example[5]: Consider

$$H(s) = \frac{1}{(s+1)\{(s+2)^2+1\}}$$

whose poles are -1 and $-2 \pm j$.

Since the eigenvalues of any 3×3 matrix $A \in C$ are constrained in the shaded area of Figure 3, $H(s)$ does *not* have a 3-dimensional realization. However, if we add the poles -2 and -3, then it has a realization of dimension 5.

$$A = \begin{pmatrix} -2 & 0 & 0 & 0 & 0 \\ 1 & -2 & 0 & 0 & 1 \\ 1 & 1 & -2 & 0 & 0 \\ 0 & 0 & 1 & -2 & 0 \\ 0 & 0 & 0 & 1 & -2 \end{pmatrix}, \quad b = \begin{pmatrix} 1 \\ 0 \\ 0 \\ 0 \\ 0 \end{pmatrix}, \quad c = \begin{pmatrix} 0 \\ 0 \\ 0 \\ 0 \\ 1 \end{pmatrix}.$$

Thus this is an example in which the minimum dimension is strictly greater than the degree of $H(s)$. Note that this realization is controllable but not observable.

We can show that a system function of this kind has a certain generic property. Note that $H(s)$, a strictly proper rational function of degree n, has $2n$ coefficients, and $H(s)$ corresponds to a $2n$-dimensional vector consisting of these coefficients in a one-to-one manner. Therefore, we can define the metric $\rho(H(s), G(s))$ between $H(s)$ and $G(s)$ by the distance between corresponding vectors in R^{2n}.

Theorem 6 : Suppose that $H(s)$ is a strictly proper rational function of degree n, and it has no n-dimensional C-realizations. Then, there is a positive number $\delta > 0$ such that $G(s)$ has no n-dimensional C-realizations whenever $\rho(H(s), G(s)) < \delta$.

Proof : This is shown by contradiction. Suppose that for any large $k > k_0$, there is a $G_k(s)$ of degree n such that $\rho(H(s), G_k(s)) \leq 1/k$ and $G_k(s)$ have an n-dimensional C-realization $(A_k, b_k, c_k, \alpha_k)$. Here b_k and c_k are unit vectors; hence, they are uniformly bounded. It can be shown that A_k is uniformly bounded by the fact that A_k satisfies Eqs. 3 and 4, and by the fact that trace(A_k), a coefficient of the denominator polynomial of $G_k(s)$, is uniformly bounded, since $G_k(s) \mapsto H(s)$ as $k \to \infty$. Also, α_k is uniformly bounded, since $G_k(s) \mapsto H(s)$. Thus, we may assume that $(A_k, b_k, c_k, \alpha_k) \mapsto (A, b, c, \alpha)$ as $k \to \infty$. Here, it can be shown that $A \in C$, b and c are unit vectors, and that α is a positive number. Thus, $\lim_{k \to \infty} G_k(s) = H(s) = \alpha \cdot c^T(sI - A)^{-1}b$ and $H(s)$, therefore, has an n-dimensional realization (A, b, c, α). This is a contradiction.

Example and Theorem 1 together imply that there is a system function $H(s)$ such that $H(s)$ itself and any other $G(s)$ near $H(s)$ do not have a controllable and observable C-realization. This indicates that we must be careful when determining the number of compartments because the number is not necessarily equal to the McMillan degree of system functions. For example, suppose I/O data were obtained from a nearly uncontrollable and/or unobservable compartmental system, and suppose we had a reduced system function $H(s)$ by eliminating the nearly uncontrollable and/or unobservable modes. Then $H(s)$ may have no C-realization with a degree equal to the McMillan degree of $H(s)$. Such a case does not occur when we are concerned with DP functions of tree-compartmental systems, since the reduced DP functions are also tree-realizable with dimensions equal to the McMillan degree of reduced DP functions.

4. CONCLUDING REMARKS

The realization problem of linear time-invariant compartmental systems has been considered, specifically, realizability conditions and minimal realizations. Concerning the realizability conditions, it seems difficult to obtain a complete answer thereto at this stage. A closely related mathematical problem is the so-called *inverse eigenvalue problem* : the problem of obtaining a necessary and sufficient condition for a set of complex (or real) numbers to be the spectrum of a non-negative matrix. This problem is also a difficult one and only partial answers are obtained. With regard to the characterization of minimal realizations as well as minimal dimensions, some attempts have been reported [10-12], in which the discretized compartmental system is considered and the problems are discussed in detail through convex cone analysis.

REFERENCES

1. Jacquez, J.A.: *Compartmental Analysis in Biology and Medicine*. Amsterdam, The Netherlands, Elsevier, 1972.
2. Schoenfeld, R.L. & Berman, M.: An electrical network analogy for isotope kinetics. *IRE National Convension Record,* Pt. 4, 84/89, 1957.
3. Hearon, J.Z.: Theorems on linear systems, *Ann. N.Y. Acad. Sci.* 108 : 36-67, 1963.
4. Rubinow, S.I. & Winzer, A.: Compartmental analysis : An inverse problem. *Math. Biosci.* 11 : 203-247, 1971.
5. Maeda, H., Kodama, S. & Kajiya, F.: Compartmental system analysis : Realization of a class of linear systems with physical constraints, *IEEE Trans. CAS-24* : 3-14, 1977.
6. Kalman, R.E.: Mathematical description of linear dynamical systems, *SIAM J. Control* 1 : 152-192, 1963.
7. Maeda, H.: System theoretical considerations for compartment analysis -transfer functions of catenary systems-(unpublished note).
8. Maeda, H., Kodama, S. & Kajiya, F.: System theoretical considerations for compartmental analysis -transfer functions of mamillary systems-, *Trans. IECE Japan,* 59-D : 347-354, 1976 (in Japanese).
9. Berman, A. & Plemmons, R.J.: *Nonnegative Matrices in the Mathematical Sciences.* Academic Press, New York, 1979.
10. Maeda, H. & Kodama, S.: Reachability, observability and realizability of linear systems with positive constraints. *Trans. IECE Japan,* 63-A : 688-694, 1930 (in Japanese).
11. Maeda, H. & Kodama, S.:Positive realization of difference equation. *IEEE Trans. CAS* 28 : 39-47, 1981.
12. Nieuwenhuis, J.W.: About nonnegative realizations. *System & Control Letters* 1 : 283-287, 1982.

PART TWO

5
RADIOCARDIOGRAPHY

Akina Hirakawa, Kotaro Minato and Michiyoshi Kuwahara

1. INTRODUCTION

In this section, we deal with a mass transport process in the blood circulatory system as an example of compartmental analysis, and show the compartmental model thereof as well as some clinical results.

2. COMPARTMENTAL MODEL

With the recent progress in radioisotope measuring devices and techniques, radiocardiography has become widely used as a method for the quantification of cardiac output, with the application of the indicator dilution method. The procedure for radiocardiography involves an injection of nondiffusible radioisotope, such as 131-I labeled human serum albumin (RIHSA), into a peripheral vein, recording a double-peaked time-activity curve (radiocardiogram, RCG) by a scintillation counter placed over the precordial region, and calibrating the concentration of radioisotope in the heart after it has been completely mixed in the circulatory system.

As the radiocardiogram shows the movement of the injected radioisotope in the heart, a compartmental model of the process can be developed as shown in Figure 1. The radioisotope is injected into the peripheral vein to simplify radiocardiography and make the procedure a safe one. Therefore, models of the injection process and the transport of radioisotope from the injection site to the right heart are pertinent. The four compartments are the right heart, pulmonary circulation (lungs), left

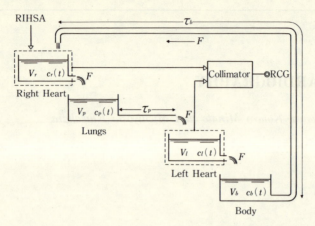

Fig. 1. Simplified model of the transport process in a circulatory system.

heart, and systemic circulation (body), and there are two transport delays, one for the pulmonary and one for the systemic circulation. In Figure 1, subscripts i, r, p, l and b denote the injection compartment, right heart, lungs, left heart and body respectively. V [ml] is the equivalent mean volume of each mixing chamber and $c(t)$ [μCi/ml] is the concentration of radioisotope in each compartment at time t. Transport delays in the lungs and the body are represented by τ_p and τ_b, respectively, and the radiocardiogram is considered to be proportional to the total amount of radioisotope in the right and left hearts.

Assuming the flow-rate of blood is constant and using as an example of a septal defect that results in an intracardiac shunt flow from the left to the right heart according to pressure differences, mathematical expressions of the transport processes of the injected radioisotope (RI) in these compartments are as follows:

(a) the injection compartment:

$$\left. \begin{aligned} & V_i \frac{dc_i(t)}{dt} = i(t) - F_i c_i(t), \\ & i(t) = \begin{cases} I/\tau, & 0 \leq t \leq \tau, \\ 0, & \tau < t, \end{cases} \\ & \int_0^\tau i(t) dt = I, \end{aligned} \right\} \quad (1)$$

where

I : total amount of injected radioisotope [μCi],
$i(t)$: injection rate [μCi/s],
τ : injection time [s],
F_i : blood flow rate in the injection compartment [ml/s].
(b) right heart:

$$V_r \frac{dc_r(t)}{dt} = F_i c_i(t) + (1-k)F c_b(t-\tau_b) + kF c_l(t) - F c_r(t), \quad (2)$$

where F is the mean blood flow rate in units of [ml/s], i.e., the cardiac output in the normal state, k represents the ratio of the shunt flow rate to the mean blood flow rate, and $F_i \ll F$.

(c) lungs:

$$V_p \frac{dc_p(t)}{dt} = F c_r(t) - F c_p(t). \quad (3)$$

(d) left heart:

$$V_l \frac{dc_l(t)}{dt} = F c_p(t-\tau_p) - F c_l(t). \quad (4)$$

(e) body:

$$V_b \frac{dc_b(t)}{dt} = (1-k)F c_l(t) - (1-k)F c_b(t), \quad (5)$$

where initial conditions are as follows:
$c_i(0)=0$,
$c_r(0)=0$,
$c_l(0)=0$,
$c_p(t)=0, \quad -\tau_p < t \leq 0$,
$c_b(t)=0, \quad -\tau_b < t \leq 0$.

Assuming that the radiocardiogram consists of counting rates from the right and left hearts at the same counting efficiency γ and that the counting rate from the background can be neglected, the radiocardiogram can be represented by

$$r(t) = \gamma [V_r c_r(t) + V_l c_l(t)]. \quad (6)$$

The actual radiocardiogram should be recorded under the same conditions as this theoretical one so that a reasonable comparison can be made between them.

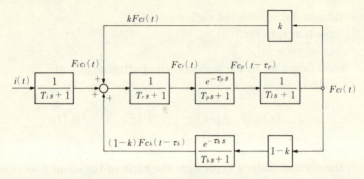

Fig. 2. Block diagram representation of the transport process in a circulatory system.

A block diagram representation of the transport process in the circulatory system can be obtained as shown in Figure 2 by calculating the Laplace transforms of Eq. 1 to Eq. 5. Each compartment, namely, the injection compartment, right heart, lungs, left heart and body, is represented by a block with a respective transfer function.

Time constants, T's, in the block diagram are as follows:

$$T_r = V_r/F,\ T_p = V_p/F,\ T_l = V_l/F,\ T_b = V_b/(1-k)F,\ T_i = V_i/F_i. \quad (7)$$

Time constants of the injection compartment, right heart, and left heart give the mean transit times of these compartments. On the other hand, the mean transit times of lungs and body can be represented by $T_p + \tau_p$ and $T_b + \tau_b$, respectively.

Values for these parameters of the block diagram can be determined by the parameter estimation procedure through the curve fitting between the actually observed and the simulated radiocardiograms. These values for the parameters correspond to the rate of intracardiac shunt k and the mean transit times of four compartments.

On the other hand, the mean concentration of radioisotope in the equilibrium state, $c(\infty)$, can be represented by

$$c(\infty) = I/V, \quad (8)$$

where V is the total circulating blood volume. The following equation is then obtained:

$$\begin{aligned}Fc(\infty) &= I/(V/F) \\ &= I/[T_r + T_p + \tau_p + T_l + (1-k)(T_b + \tau_b)]. \quad (9)\end{aligned}$$

The mean concentration of radioisotope in the equilibrium state can be measured by a well-type scintillation counter. All values for the parameters in the right-hand side of Eq. 9 can be determined through the curve-fitting procedure, using an analog computer. Then, Eq. 9 gives the mean rate for blood flow in the left heart, F, i.e., the cardiac output.

3. CLINICAL RESULTS

Figures 3 to 6 show some clinical simulation results for various patients.

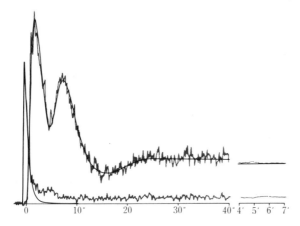

Fig. 3. RCG and simulation results for a normal subject. Simulation data (49-year-old male): Circulating blood volume: 2.65 liters/m^2, heart rate: 100. Mean transit time: right heart 2.1 sec, lung 4.2 sec, left heart 2.3 sec, body 25.7 sec. Cardiac index: 4.64 liters/min/m^2. Right heart volume: 161 ml/m^2, left heart volume: 176 ml/m^2. Pulmonary blood volume: 326 ml/m^2, blood volume of body: 1991 ml/m^2.

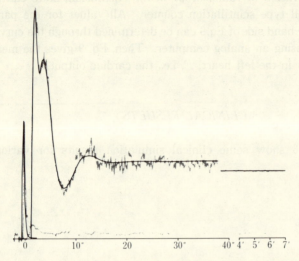

Fig. 4. RCG and simulation results of a patient with hyperthyroidism. Simulation data (15-year-old female): Circulating blood volume: 2.75 liters/m^2, heart rate 112. Mean transit time: right heart 1.2 sec, lung 1.4 sec, left heart 1.1 sec, body 12.5 sec. Cardiac index: 10.2 liters/min/m^2. Right heart volume: 201 ml/m^2, left heart volume: 185 ml/m^2. Pulmonary blood volume: 230 ml/m^2, blood volume of body: 2034 ml/m^2.

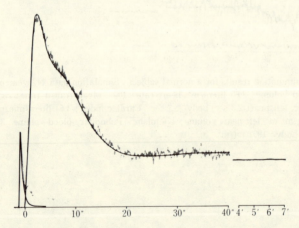

Fig. 5. RCG and simulation results for a patient with right heart failure and bronchial asthma. Simulation data (47-year-old male): Circulating blood volume: 2.98 liters/m^2, heart rate: 89. Mean transit time: right heart 7.7 sec, lung 5.5 sec, left heart 2.0 sec, body 44.6 sec. Cardiac index: 2.99 liters/min/m^2. Right heart volume: 383 ml/m^2, left heart volume: 100 ml/m^2. Pulmonary blood volume: 274 ml/m^2, blood volume of body: 2221 ml/m^2.

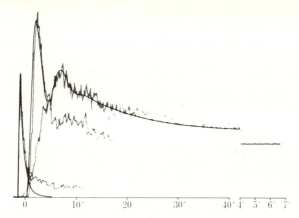

Fig. 6. RCG and simulation results for a patient with atrial septal defect and pulmonary hypertension. Simulation data (21-year-old male) : Circulating blood volume : 3.19 liters/m², heart rate : 67. Mean transit time : right heart 1.7 sec, lung 4.1 sec, left heart 0.5 sec, body 47.5 sec. Pulmonary blood flow rate (PBF) : 20.5 liters/min, systemic blood flow rate (SBF) : 4.10 liters/min. L-R shunt : 16.4 liters/min (80 % of PBF). Cardiac index : 2.44 liters/min/m². Right heart volume : 339 ml/m², left heart volume : 94 ml/m². Pulmonary blood volume : 823 ml/m², blood volume of body : 1929 ml/m². Cardiac catheterization data (heart rate : 67) : Pulmonary blood flow rate (PBF) : 26.5 liters/min, systemic blood flow rate (SBF) : 4.40 liters/min. L-R shunt : 22.1 liters/min (83 % of PBF). Cardiac index : 2.60 liters/min/m².

REFERENCES

1. Kuwahara, M., Hirakawa, A., Kinoshita, M. et al.: Analysis of radiocardiogram by analog computer simulation. *Int. J. Biomed. Eng.* 1 : 13-21, 1972.
2. Minato, K., Kuwahara, M., Yonekura, Y. et al.: Parameter estimation of radiocardiogram using a minicomputer. *Automatica* 15 : 521-529, 1979.

6
HYDROGEN GAS CLEARANCE METHOD FOR REGIONAL MYOCARDIAL BLOOD FLOW

Masahiko Kinoshita

1. INTRODUCTION

The hydrogen gas clearance technique has been applied to the measurement of blood flow in various types of tissue such as brain[1], heart[2], intestine[3], pancreas[4], spinal cord[5], uterus[6], dental pulp[7], capital femoral epiphysis[8], skeletal muscle[1], kidney[1], tongue[9], and bone marrow[10]. The method by which the local tissue blood flow is measured in an organ of two or more compartments with different blood flows has been reported using the inert gas desaturation curve, but considerable error in the calculated mean flow may be expected if the flow rate varies widely in the different compartments of one organ. Regional myocardial blood flow (RMBF) disturbances have recently been demonstrated in clinical cardiology using the Gamma camera and computer[11]. The precordial ^{133}Xe clearance technique may be the only clinical method currently available for estimating RMBF quantitatively[12]. However, with the precordial method, transmyocardial blood flow is not separated accurately. The tracer microsphere technique, therefore, is the only method that can be used effectively to measure RMBF properly. It is the most accurate method currently available for the measurement of transmural blood flow[13], but repeated measurements can be taken on only six occasions, because the maximum number of different isotopes that can be used is six. On the other hand, frequent measurements of tissue blood flow can be taken by the hydrogen gas washout method, whereby hydrogen concentrations in tissue are measured continuously through a platinum electrode inserted into the tissue. This chapter also deals with the validity of the hydrogen method compared with the tracer microsphere technique. Furthermore, application of the hydrogen method to see the effects of coronary artery stenosis, cardiovascular drug administration, intramyocardial pressure, and heart rate on RMBF will be described.

2. METHOD

2.1 PRINCIPLE OF HYDROGEN DETERMINATION

This method is one in which the hydrogen gas washout curve is obtained by readings with the platinum electrode embedded in the tissue after the inhalation of hydrogen gas[1]. The hydrogen gas in the tissue is oxidized to produce the reaction $H_2 = 2H + 2e^-$ on the surface of the platinum, setting up a concentration gradient between tissue and platinum electrode. As a result a diffusion current linearly proportional to the concentration gradient is generated at the electrode. The current is in the order of 10^{-8} ampere and can be converted to voltage amplified by a high-gain amplifier. The derivation of the equation for determining RMBF is largely based on Kety's equation, which comes from the Fick principle. The amount (dQ_i) of hydrogen gas accumulated in tissue supplied by a homogeneous and constant blood flow (F ml/sec) in time dt is:

$$dQ_i = (C_a - C_{vi}) \cdot F dt, \qquad (1)$$

where C_a is the arterial concentration, and C_{vi} the venous concentration of hydrogen in the tissue. If C_i is the concentration in tissue with volume W, then Eq. 1 will read:

$$W dC_i = (C_a - C_{vi}) \cdot F dt. \qquad (2)$$

When the diffusion between hydrogen gas and tissue occurs instantaneously, with λ as the tissue/blood partition coefficient for hydrogen, the following equation will be derived:

$$W dC_i = (C_a - C_i/\lambda) \cdot F dt. \qquad (3)$$

If the hydrogen gas is rapidly removed from the lung when gas inhalation stops, C_a will be equal to zero.

$$dC_i/C_i = -F/\lambda W \, dt. \qquad (4)$$

Integration of Eq. 4 from $t=0$ to $t=t$ yields

$$C_i = C_{io} e^{-kt}, \qquad (5)$$

where $k = F/\lambda W$.

The value of k is calculated from the monoexponential curve using a desk calculator. Since, according to Aukland[1], λ is equal to 1, k can be converted to flow per unit volume (F/W) expressed in ml/min/g.

2.2 MEASURING CIRCUIT AND PLATINUM ELECTRODE

The electrode was made from platinum wire, 0.1 mm in diameter, insulated with epoxy resin, leaving a 1-mm-long uninsulated segment. Before use, electrolysis, in a 5% platinum chloride solution, deposited platinum black on the surface of the uninsulated segment of the electrode. The elecrodes were then sewn into the myocardium. The circuit consisted of an amplifier and the head of the amplifier, which were placed next to the experimental dog. The platinum electrodes were polarized with a potential of +0.3 V relative to an Ag/AgCl electrode inserted into the subcutaneous tissue of the thorax.

2.3 RECIRCULATION OF HYDROGEN GAS

The hydrogen gas should not be allowed to recirculate when applying Kety's equation for measuring tissue blood flow. However, it is difficult to clear hydrogen gas from the pulmonary circulation in one passage through the lungs, even if the blood/gas partition coefficient is as small as 0.018. Aukland[1] reported that when hydrogen respiration ceased, it took 40 to 50 sec before the concentration of hydrogen in arterial blood fell below 10% of its initial concentration. This experience showed that in most cases the arterial concentration declined to 10% of the initial concentration after 40 sec. Arterial hypoxia may occur with prolonged hydrogen gas inhalation. Tamura[14] suggested that 3 to 5 min of inhalation would be suitable. However, in this study a 1-min inhalation provided a good hydrogen gas clearance curve from the myocardium[15].

2.4 PROCEDURES

Adult mongrel dogs, weighing 10 to 24 kg, were anesthetized using pentobarbital sodium, intubated by an endotracheal tube, and thoracotomized through the 5th intercostal space. The catheters were placed in the left ventricular cavity and aorta, respectively. Hydrogen gas was administered at a flow rate of 1 l/min for about 1 min through a side tube attached to the endotracheal tube. Four electrodes were sewn into the subendocardium (END) and subepicardium (EPI), in the regions supplied by the left circumflex and the anterior descending arteries, respectively. The intramyocardial electrocardiograms were taken using platinum electrodes to make sure that the electrodes were properly placed and to judge the extent of myocardial ischemia.

3. VALIDATION OF THE METHOD

3.1 LINEARITY OF THE SYSTEM

Using a test chamber with a magnetic stirrer, the linearity of the system was examined. Repeated injections of a known amount of hydrogen-saturated saline into a test chamber containing 100 ml of hydrogen-free saline, produced a step-wise decline in hydrogen concentration in that chamber[15]. The recorded response relative to hydrogen concentration gave an excellent linear response, with a correlation coefficient of 0.99.

3.2 REPEATABILITY

Two repeated measurements for the clearance curve were taken 15 min apart in 11 different dogs. The measurements showed a correlation coefficient of 0.91, ranging from ±15% of a line of unity. In addition, 10 successive measurements in one dog gave a coefficient of variation of 6.3%. Thus, the more than 10% difference in flow rate for different measurements was thought to be significant.

3.3 COMPARISON WITH TRACER MICROSPHERE METHOD

The radiomicrosphere technique is the most accurate method currently available for measuring RMBF. Measurements were taken by the microsphere and the hydrogen gas clearance method simultaneously in 4 dogs in which 14 measurements were compared. As shown in Figure 1, there was a good correlation between the RMBF obtained by hydrogen gas clearance and that by the radioactive microsphere method. However, the hydrogen method gave an average value 9% lower than that of the microsphere method. Not many reports have been published comparing the hydrogen clearance and microsphere methods for measuring RMBF[16]. However, LaMorgese[17] showed that values recorded for cerebral blood flow using the hydrogen method tended to be lower than those recorded with the microsphere method. Meyer and Path[7] reported that blood flows obtained with 15μ microspheres and hydrogen averaged 0.60 and 0.20 ml/min/g in the dental pulp of dogs. They concluded that the blood flows obtained using the

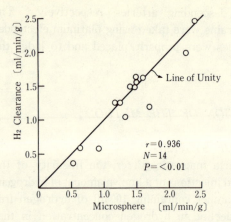

Fig. 1. RMBFs obtained using hydrogen clearance and radioactive microsphere methods.

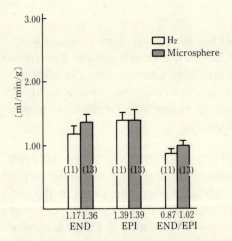

Fig. 2. Normal values for RMBF obtained using the hydrogen clearance and radioactive microsphere method. Figures in parentheses denote the number of cases.

hydrogen method were significantly lower than those using the 15μ microsphere method, which provided the most accurate results. These findings suggest that the hydrogen method underestimates pulp blood flow because of arterial-venous shunting. Another reason for the underestimation may be the recirculation of hydrogen gas inhaled during respiration. A third reason may be inhomogeneity of flow in the area surrounding the electrode.

The hydrogen clearance curve mainly reflects the slower components, and the average flow will be underestimated in the area with inhomogeneous flow.

Normal values for RMBF obtained by hydrogen gas clearance and the tracer microsphere methods were compared for the area supplied by the left anterior descending artery. The normal RMBFs by the hydrogen method were 1.17 ± 0.14(SEM) ml/min/g in END and 1.39 ± 0.12 ml/min/g in EPI; the ratio of END/EPI blood flow was 0.87 ± 0.08, denoting a significant decrease in END blood flow. In contrast, there was no significant difference between END and EPI blood flow with the tracer method (Fig. 2). In general, reports on the use of the tracer microsphere method showed an END preponderance over EPI blood flow[18], whereas those in which the hydrogen clearance method was used showed that EPI blood flow tended to be higher than the END[15,19].

3.4 PROBLEMS OF THE HYDROGEN GAS CLEARANCE METHOD

A number of factors may preclude correct estimations with the hydrogen gas clearance method. According to Aukland[1], a change in temperature, pH, pO_2 and ascorbic acid *in vivo* may introduce some errors. Direct insertion of a platinum electrode may injure the tissue surrounding the electrode. Microscopic studies of the effect of electrode insertion on myocardial tissue showed only very slight bleeding and polynuclear infiltration around the electrode[15]. Although it is also suggested that the smaller the electrode, the less the degree of tissue injury, a diameter of 100 μm may be the most appropriate for measuring myocardial blood flow. Since the hydrogen clearance curve mainly reflects the slower components, the average flow will be underestimated in the region with inhomogeneous flow. Aukland[1] suggested that the slope method is misleading when a flow rate above 1.50 ml/min/g is to be determined and that the area integrated between the arterial and tissue concentration curves will reflect the mean flow rate more accurately than the slope method. Most hydrogen curves from the myocardium show a monoexponential slope but some fit a biexponential pattern. A comparison between RMBF values calculated by an initial slope method with one-compartment analysis and by the stochastic method of height over area is shown in Figure 3. There was no consistent difference between the two methods, indicating the slope method can accurately reflect flow rate.

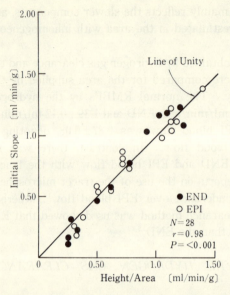

Fig. 3. The comparison between an initial slope method and the stochastic method of height over area.

4. APPLICATION OF THE HYDROGEN GAS CLEARANCE METHOD

4.1 THE EFFECT OF CORONARY ARTERY STENOSIS ON RMBF

Coronary stenosis produced a preferential END ischemia, indicating that the inner layers of the ventricle are more severely compromised than the outer layers. This evidence is mostly derived from data obtained using the tracer microsphere method. In the present study, gradual stenosis of the left anterior descending artery produced a gradual decrease in regional END and EPI blood flows, being slightly more pronounced in the former. Intramyocardial ST-segment elevation occurred at an average flow rate of 0.32 ml/min/g for END and 0.74 ml/min/g for EPI, denoting a decrease of 33% and 64% in END and EPI relative to values recorded prior to the coronary stenosis[24]. Going further into the relationship between ST-segment elevation and RMBF, epicardial ST-segment elevation began to occur at an END flow rate of less than 0.50 ml/min/g. There was no clear relationship between EPI blood flow and ST-segment elevation, since ST-segment elevation took place at an EPI blood flow higher than 0.50 ml/min/g, that is, EPI ST-segment elevation reflected as END blood flow. The present study demonstrated that the ratio of END to EPI started to decrease when coronary perfusion pressure decreased to 77 mmHg, and that ST segment elevation occurred at a coronary pressure of 45 mmHg. Therefore, it can be concluded that the autoregulatory reserve of END is smaller than that of EPI.

4.2 RELATIONSHIP BETWEEN INTRAMYOCARDIAL PRESSURE AND RMBF

The consequences of the *intramyocardial pressure* across the myocardial wall in diastole to the RMBF have not been fully explored[20]. Intramyocardial pressure was measured using a MIKRO-TIP catheter pressure transducer with a hypodermic needle (Millar Instruments, Inc.)[21] The sensor was placed 5 mm apart from the tip of the needle. The dimensions of the sensing portion of the probe were $1 \times 1.6 \times 2$ mm. The needle probe was inserted at an angle of about 45° directly into the wall of the left ventricle and positioned at a depth of 9 mm for END and 4 mm for EPI in the free wall. RMBF showed 0.67 and 0.87 ml/min/g in END and EPI, respectively, for the control state. Following an infusion of dextran 40, left ventricular end-diastolic pressure increased from 2.9 mmHg to 40.6

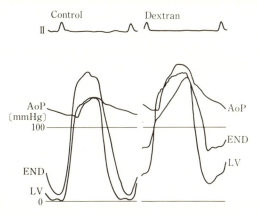

Fig. 4. Intramyocardial pressure in subendocardium (END), left ventricular pressure (LV), and aortic pressure (AoP) for control and after dextran infusion.

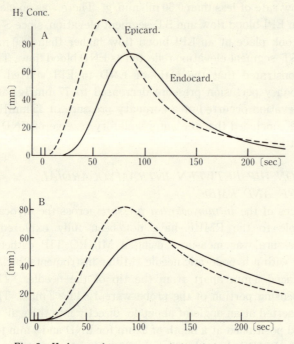

Fig. 5. Hydrogen clearance curve before (A) and after (B) dextran infusion.

mmHg, and end-diastolic intramyocardial pressure increased from 9.9 mmHg to 78.2 mmHg (Fig. 4). At this time, the RMBF was 0.46 and 0.69 ml/min/g in END and EPI, respectively. The ratio of END to EPI decreased from 0.77 in the control to 0.67 after dextran infusion. Thus, an increasing preload elevates diastolic intramyocardial pressure, which decreases END more than EPI blood flow (Fig. 5).

4.3 EFFECTS OF NITRATE ON RMBF

Myocardial ischemia with or without angina will result from an imbalance between myocardial oxygen demand and supply. Since nitrate has been used as an antianginal drug for over 100 years, this drug must restore the balance in the ischemic myocardium either by increasing myocardial blood flow or by decreasing oxygen consumption. To examine its effect on RMBF, isosorbide dinitrate was given intravenously to dogs with coronary artery stenosis in which ischemia was augmented by a preload increase. As shown in Figure 6, isosorbide dinitrate administration significantly in-

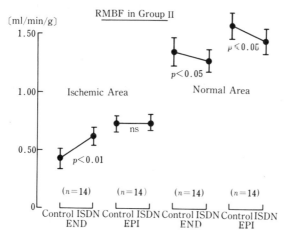

Fig. 6. Effect of isosorbide dinitrate on RMBF.

creased END blood flow but not EPI blood flow, in the ischemic area improving the ratio of END to EPI blood flow in the ischemic area. In the nonischemic area, END and EPI blood flow decreased significantly, indicating that the myocardium required less oxygen. ST-segment elevation was also improved in dogs with (Group II) and without (Group I) a preload increase after isosorbide dinitrate administration[22]. Therefore, the mechanism of the antianginal action of nitrate may be assumed to be as follows: venodilatory action of nitrate leads to a diminution in preload which induces a decrease in left ventricular end-diastolic pressure and END tissue pressure. As a result END capillaries in the ischemic region no longer collapsed. A decrease in RMBF in the non-ischemic region reflects a decrease in myocardial oxygen consumption.

4.4 EFFECT OF PROPRANOLOL ON RMBF

Although propranolol decreases total coronary blood flow, it redistributes the RMBF from normal to ischemic myocardium, improving the ratio of END to EPI blood flow (Fig. 7). The present study demonstrated that propranolol increased the END blood flow in ischemic areas, but decreased END and EPI blood flow in normal areas, thereby improving the ratio of END to EPI blood flow in the ischemic area. The effect of propranolol will be, in part, secondary to its bradycardic action of decreasing oxygen demand, leading to an improvement in the supply-demand ratio[23].

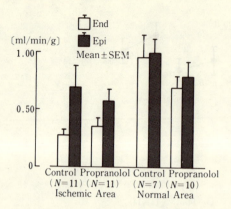

Fig. 7. Effect of propranolol on RMBF.

5. CONCLUSION

The hydrogen clearance method is, at least theoretically, an established method for measuring RMBF. The clearance curve can be measured repeatedly with a wire-type platinum electrode implanted in the myocardium. The repeatability and reliability of the method were ascertained by comparing it with the radioactive tracer method, which is thought to be the most accurate procedure currently available. The hydrogen clearance method can be applied to studies of the coronary circulation and of the effects of various types of cardiovascular drugs on RMBF.

ACKNOWLEDGMENTS

The author wishes to thank Drs. Yukio Takayama and Seiichi Kawakita for encouragement in performing this research, Messrs. Mikio Nakagawa and Hiroshi Okuno for their technical assistance, and Mr. Leslie Brizzak for preparing the manuscript of this chapter.

REFERENCES

1 Aukland, K., Bower, B.F. & Berliner, B.W.: Measurement of local blood flow with hydrogen

gas. *Circ. Res.* 14 : 164-187, 1964.
2. Aukland, K., Kiil, F., Kjekshus, J. et al. : Local myocardial blood flow measured by hydrogen polarography : Distribution and effect of hypoxia. *Acta Physiol. Scand.* 70 : 99-111, 1967.
3. Mishima, Y., Shigematsu, H., Horie, Y. et al. : Measurement of local blood flow of the intestine by hydrogen clearance method : Experimental study. *Jpn. J. Surg.* 9 : 63-70, 1979.
4. Nagata, K., Watanabe, Y. & Adachi, J. : Pancreatic local blood flow in experimental acute pancreatitis. *Jpn. J. Digestive Organs* 76 : 2054, 1979 (in Japanese).
5. Senter, H.J., Burgess, D.H. & Metzler, J. : An improved technique for measurement of spinal cord blood flow. *Brain Res.* 149 : 197-203, 1978.
6. Klingenberg, I. : The effect of radium on blood flow in the human uterine cervix measured by local hydrogen clearance. *Acta Obstet. Gynecol. Scand.* 53 : 7-11, 1974.
7. Meyer, M.W. & Path, M.G. : Blood flow in the dental pulp of dogs determined by hydrogen polarography and radioactive microsphere methods. *Arch. Oral Biol.* 24 : 601-605, 1979.
8. Schoenecker, P.L., Bitch, M. & Witeside, L.A. : The acute effect of position of immobilization on capital femoral epiphyseal blood flow. A quantitative study using the hydrogen washout technique. *J.Bone Joint Surg.* 60 : 899-904, 1978.
9. Fazekas, P., Zosch, E. & Harsing, L. : Regional blood flow and collateral circulation of the tongue in the dog studied by hydrogen polarography. *Oral Surg* 46 · 755-758, 1978.
10. Whiteside, L.A., Lesker, P.A. & Simmons, D.J. : Measurement of regional bone marrow blood flow in the rabbit using the hydrogen washout technique. *Clin. Orthop.* 122 : 340-346, 1977.
11. Schad, N. & Nichel, O. : Detection of regional flow disturbances with the Gamma-Camera. *The pathophysiology of myocardial perfusion.* ed. by W. Schaper, Elsevier/North-Holland Biomedical Press, Amsterdam, New York, Oxford, pp. 43-92, 1979.
12. Ross, R.S., Ueda, K., Lichtlen, P.R. et al. : Measurement of myocardial blood flow in animals and man by selective injection of radioactive inert gas into the coronary arteries. *Circ. Res.* 15 : 28-41, 1964.
13. Wagner, Jr., H.N., Rhodes, B.A., Sasaki, J. et al. : Studies of the circulation with radioactive microspheres. *Invest. Radiol.* 4 : 374-386, 1969.
14. Tamura, A., Asano, T., Tak, Y. et al. : Measurement of cerebral blood flow with hydrogen clearance method : Technique and a comparative study with the venous out-flow method. *Nohshinkei* 30 : 47-54, 1978 (in Japanese).
15. Kinoshita, M., Takayama, Y. & Kawakita, S. : Measurement of regional myocardial blood flow with hydrogen clearance method. *J. Jap. Coll. Angiol.* 21 : 183-188, 1981 (in Japanese).
16. Gross, G.J. & Winbury, M.M. : Betaadrenergic blockade on intramyocardial distribution of coronary blood flow. *J. Pharmcol. Exp. Ther.* 187 : 451-464, 1973.
17. LaMorgese, J., Fein, J.M. & Shulman, K. : Polarographic and microsphere analysis of ultraregional cerebral blood flow rates in the cat. In *Blood flow and metabolism in the brain.* Harper, A.M, Jennet, W.B., Mitler, J.D., Rowan, J.O. (Eds) London, Churchill, Livingstone, pp. 73-78, 1975.
18. Buckberg, B.D., Luch, J.C, Payne, D.B. et al. : Some sources of errors in measuring regional blood flow with radioactive microspheres. *J.Appl. Physiol.* 31 : 598-604, 1971.
19. Maruyama, Y. : Studies on regional myocardial blood flow. *Tohhoku Ishi* 85 : 217-252, 1971 (in Japanese).
20. Kjekshus, J.K. : Mechanism for flow distribution in normal and ischemic myocardium during increased ventricular preload in the dog. *Circ. Res.* 33 : 489-499, 1973.
21. Stein, P.D., Sabbah, H.S., Margilli, M. et al. : Comparison of the distribution of intramyocardial pressure across the canine left ventricular wall in the beating heart during diastole and in the arrested heart. *Circ. Res.* 47 : 258-267, 1980.
22. Takayama, Y., Kinoshita, M. & Kawakita, S. : Effect of isosorbide dinitrate on regional

myocardial blood flow during increased ventricular preload in the dog. *J. Jpn. Coll. Angiol.* 21 : 351-357, 1971 (in Japanese).

23 Winbury, M.M. & Howe, B.B.: Stenosis: Regional myocardial ischemia and reserve in ischemic myocardium and antianginal drugs, edited by M.M. Winbury and Y. Abiko. Raven Press, New York, pp. 55-76, 1979.

24 Takayama, Y., Kinoshita, M. & Kawakita, S.: Vertical (END to EPI) Extension of myocardial ischemia following multistage coronary stenosis in the dog. *J. Jpn. Coll. Angiol.* 22 : 67-74, 1982 (in Japanese).

7
TURNOVER OF SERUM ENZYMES AND ITS APPLICATION TO QUANTITATIVE ASSESSMENT OF MYOCARDIAL INFARCT SIZE

Michitoshi Inoue, Masatsugu Hori and Hiroshi Abe

1. TURNOVER OF TISSUE ENZYMES

1.1 RELEASE OF TISSUE ENZYMES INTO THE CIRCULATION

Over the past two decades a large number of serum enzyme tests have been used to detect tissue damage in various diseases. Since high serum enzyme activity reflects the release of appropriate enzymes from damaged tissue into the circulation, tissue injury can be diagnosed from serum concentrations of a particular enzyme in that tissue. Therefore, the high serum activities of aspartate transaminase (AST) and alanine transaminase (ALT) suggest liver involvement, while high creatine kinase (CK) activities imply myocardial infarction or muscular injury, since the liver is rich in the former enzymes, whereas the myocardium and skeletal muscle are rich in the latter.

Although the mechanism and time course of the release of an enzyme from a cell have not been fully clarified, increased permeability of the cell membrane either by inflammatory or ischemic processes is thought to release the enzymes in cytosol, such as AST, lactate dehydrogenase (LD), and CK[1]. In necrotic conditions, however, profound cellular damage is followed by the appearance of mitochondrial enzymes, e.g., m-AST in serum[2]. If acute tissue damage occurs, as in acute myocardial infarction or traumatic injury, the onset of enzyme release is clearly evidenced by an abrupt increase in serum enzyme activity after a certain time lag following the onset of tissue damage. Once tissue enzymes leak out of a cell, they are washed out of the intercellular space into the circulating blood through lymphatic flow and venous drainage[3]. Thus, peak serum enzyme levels should correlate with the total amount of enzyme released from the damaged tissue, if cellular injury begins simultaneously throughout the tissue.

2. REMOVAL OF ENZYMES FROM THE CIRCULATION

Although it is well known that serum enzymes are removed at different rates, either in acute hepatitis or in acute myocardial infarction, their fate is not fully understood[4]. Excretion in urine is considered to be a minor factor, except for low molecular weight enzymes such as amylase (molecular weight: about 45,000)[5]. The major mechanism whereby serum enzymes are removed may be intravascular inactivation, either by some proteolytic enzymes or by antigen-antibody reaction. Another possible mechanism is their digestion and decomposition to amino acids once they appear in the intestine[1]. However, whatever the mechanism whereby serum enzymes are removed, it seems that each has its own rate of disappearance from serum.

Figure 1 shows representative serial changes in serum enzymes in a patient with acute myocardial infarction. In all of the enzymes studied, decays in serum levels are exponential after each peak. Thus, the rate at

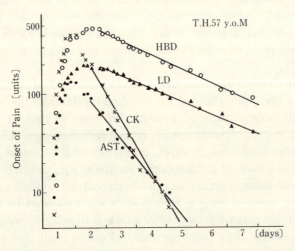

Fig. 1. Serial changes in serum enzyme activities in acute myocardial infarction [Reproduced by permission from Medical J. Osaka Univ. vol. 25, p. 169, 1975].

which each disappears from the circulation can be obtained from the slope of these decays in a semilogarithmic plot. LD and α-hydroxybutyric acid dehydrogenase (HBD) have slow, whereas CK and AST have rapid decay rates. These discrepancies in disappearance rates among the various enzymes may be very important, because the time to peak activity after the onset of acute myocardial infarction and the duration of abnormally high serum levels depend mainly on the disappearance rate of the enzyme. Therefore, serum levels of LD and HBD with slow decay rates are diagnostically useful even several days after the onset of infarction[7].

3. COMPARTMENTAL MODEL OF TURNOVER OF SERUM CREATINE KINASE IN ACUTE MYOCARDIAL INFARCTION

3.1 A COMPARTMENTAL MODEL FOR ASSESSMENT OF INFARCT SIZE FROM SERUM CK ACTIVITIES

Serum creatine kinase (CK), especially its myocardial CK-MB isoenzyme, is highly specific and sensitive. Therefore, it is helpful in the diagnosis of acute myocardial infarction[8] and widely used to detect myocardial injury. Furthermore, myocardial CK depletion has been shown to be proportional to the size of the infarct[9], the fraction of CK released from the center of an infarct being relatively constant[9,10]. Based on these findings and the mono-exponential decay of serum CK injected intravenously into conscious dogs, Shell et al. proposed a compartmental model for the kinetics of serum CK and developed a method for the quantitative assessment of infarct size from a serial determination of serum CK activities[11].

The decay in serum CK appears mono-exponential except in the initial phase in which the enzyme is probably diluted in its effective distribution space. Fortunately, its disappearance rate has not been shown to be influenced by hemodynamic changes[11]. Consequently, Shell et al. proposed the following mathematical model for calculating the size of an infarct:

$$dE(t)/dt = f(t) - K_d \cdot E(t) \quad (1)$$

$E(t)$: serum CK concentration
$f(t)$: function of appearance of myocardial CK in circulation
K_d: rate of disappearance from circulation

$$CK_r = (D.S.) \cdot \int_0^t f(t) dt \quad (2)$$

CK_r : total CK released from infarcted myocardium
$D.S.$: distribution space for CK ($0.114 \times$ body weight)

$$\text{infarct size (g)} = CK_r / K \cdot [CK_d] \tag{3}$$

K : fraction of CK lost from myocardium that appears in the CK distribution space
$[CK_d]$: CK activity depleted from 1 g of infarcted myocardium

The rationale for this model is based on the kinetics of serum CK. Instantaneous serum CK activity is regulated by the disappearance rate of CK from serum tissue into the circulation, $f(t)$ and the depleted CK from serum. The latter is proportional to the instantaneous serum activity and the rate at which it disappears from serum ($K_d \cdot E(t)$).

Serial changes in serum CK activities ($E(t)$) are obtained from their serial determinations at 1 to 4 h intervals after the onset of infarction until serum CK levels return to normal. A percutaneous catheter inserted into the antecubital vein is widely used for blood sampling. The rate at which CK activity disappears from serum can be obtained from the decay slope of ($E(t)$) using a semi-logarithmic plot. Since Norris et al.[12] reported that individual disappearance rates vary widely, a decay rate was obtained from each curve of serum CK activity in our study (modified method of Norris et al.). The total amount of CK released, i.e., integrated released CK activity $\left(\int_0^t f(t) dt \right)$ was expressed in our study as total units of CK released per milliliter of serum because the fraction of CK activity depleted from the infarcted myocardium and appearing in serum may depend on the size of the infarct. This variation could cause an error in g-equivalent infarct size.

3.2 LIMITATION OF THE FIRST-ORDER COMPARTMENTAL MODEL

Shell's method, described above, is based on a single compartmental model for the kinetics of serum CK, assuming a mono-exponential decay of serum CK activity. However, recent careful study of serum CK decay after a bolus injection of purified myocardial CK in conscious dogs has demonstrated that a double-exponential is much closer than a single-exponential fit[13]. This suggested the existence of one extravascular compartment as a CK distribution space. Therefore, a two-compartment model was proposed by Sobel et al. With this model, an extravascular compartment may play an important role in the double-exponentiality of serum CK decay; changes in CK volume in the vascular ($E_v(t)$) and extravascular ($E_e(t)$) compartments are described in the following equations, where $g(t)$ is an input function:

$$dE_v(t)/dt = \lambda_{ve}E_e(t) - (\lambda_{ev}+\lambda_v)E_v(t) + g(t)$$
$$dE_e(t)/dt = \lambda_{ev}E_v(t) - \lambda_{ve}E_e(t)$$

$\lambda_{ev}, \lambda_{ve}$: exchange rates from vascular to extravascular pool and from extravascular to vascular pool
λ_v : true rate of disappearance from the blood pool

Sobel et al. found that the parameters of a 2-compartment model obtained from the double-exponential curve provide estimates of the true rate at which serum CK disappears, which are significantly greater than the observed elimination rate. Accordingly, the total quantity of CK released, as calculated from these estimates of the true disappearance rate, was almost twice that obtained by calculations in which the observed elimination rate was used. Unfortunately, however, in patients with acute myocardial infarction the serum CK decay curve after the peak cannot be used directly to obtain parameters of the 2-compartment model. This is because the initial decay observed after a bolus injection of purified CK in animal experiments, may be masked by the continuing release of CK from the myocardium during the early decay phase. Therefore, we should apply the single compartmental model to the clinical assessment of infarct size, keeping the inherent limitations of the model in mind.

4. ESTIMATION OF INFARCT SIZE BY SERIAL SERUM CK DETERMINATION

4.1 ASSESSMENT OF EVOLUTION OF MYOCARDIAL INFARCTION

The appearance function of serum CK (the rate of release of myocardial CK into the circulation) should indicate the evolution of myocardial infarction. Therefore, whether the time required for an infarct to evolve correlated with its size and clinical symptoms was studied in 50 patients with acute myocardial infarction[14]. The relationships between ST-T segment changes, the development of abnormal Q waves, and the evolution of the infarct, were also studied in this series and in another series of 27

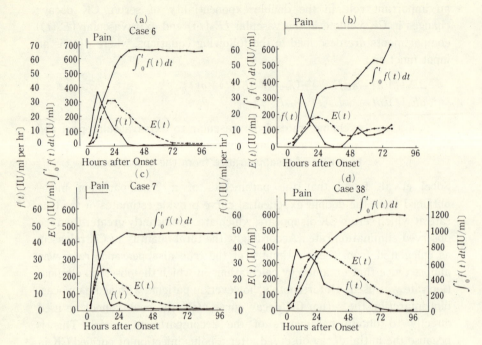

Fig. 2. Serial serum CK activities ($E(t)$), appearance function ($f(t)$), accumulated CK released ($\int_0^t f(t)dt$) and duration of chest pain in four representative cases with acute myocardial infarction [Reproduced by permission from Brit. Heart J. 42: 487, 1977].

patients[15].

Figure 2 depicts the appearance functions ($f(t)$) of CK and the duration of chest pain in four representative cases. In all cases the duration of pain corresponded to the duration of the major release of CK from the myocardium involved. The mean duration of CK release in 50 patients was 37.2±2.4 (SE) hours, after which ST-T changes in the precordial electrocardiogram stabilized. It should also be noted that the duration of CK release in patients without heart failure was significantly shorter than that in patients with heart failure, while the duration of the release correlated roughly, but significantly (r=0.67, p<0.01), with infarct size (total CK release; $\int_0^t f(t)dt$). Thus, the long duration of chest pain may suggest a large infarction, although this complaint may be largely affected by the various conditions of patients.

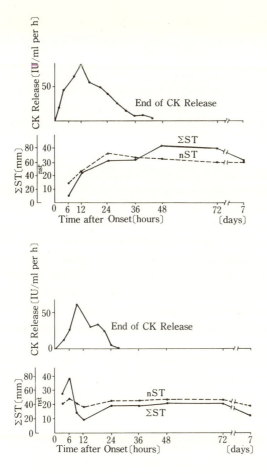

Fig. 3. Representative serial changes in CK release ($f(t)$), ΣST and nST in two patients with acute myocardial infarction [Reproduced by permission from Brit. Heart J. 42: 728, 1979].

Figure 3 shows the serial changes in CK release rates and ΣST (the sum of ST segment elevations) and nST (the number of leads showing ST segment elevation) in precordial ST mapping in two representative cases. It should be noted that in both cases ΣST and nST stabilized near the point at which the infarct had completed evolving, judging from the appearance of CK release. Moreover, the ΣST and nST obtained when release of CK had ceased, correlated closely with the total amount of CK released, i.e. infarct size, whereas values recorded on admission correlate only poorly.

The release of CK also corresponded to the amplitude of abnormal Q waves in the patients with inferior infarctions. These results indicate that the appearance function of CK release ($f(t)$) represents the evolution of myocardial infarction. The length of time over which myocardial infarction evolves in man, could usually be much longer than that in dogs, and this may encourage early therapeutic interventions such as emergency coronary angioplasty or the administration of various drugs to protect the jeopardized ischemic myocardium.

4.2 INFARCT SIZE AND CARDIAC FUNCTION

As described previously, the cumulative amount of CK released could correlate with a g-equivalent infarct size in Sobel's method. The original study in which this method was applied to man revealed that in patients who died of heart failure or who survived but manifested marked functional impairment, mean infarct size was much larger (more than three times) than in patients who survived without marked heart failure[16]. Norris et al. also reported that the total amount of CK released was greater with transmural infarction than that with subendocardial infarction, and showed a close positive correlation with clinical indices of the extent of myocardial damage[12].

We investigated the relationship between infarct size and left ventricular ejection fraction, cardiac index and left ventricular end-diastolic pressure (LVEDP) measured after the infarct had healed, in 34 patients with acute myocardial infarction[17]. A close inverse correlation (r = −0.71 in 18 patients with anterior infarction, r = −0.73 in 16 patients with inferior infarction) was observed between total CK released and ejection fraction, although the cardiac index was maintained over $2.0/min/m^2$ in almost all patients. Moreover, it is of interest that the ejection fraction in patients with anterior myocardial infarction was lower than in those with inferior myocardial infarction with comparable values of total CK released. This may indicate that left ventricular function after infarction depends on the site of the infarct.

4.3 SITE OF CORONARY NARROWING AND INFARCT SIZE IN MAN

Although the site of a coronary lesion is considered to be one of the major determinants of infarct size, this relationship in man remains to be elucidated, since histologically assessed infarct size in postmortem studies may not represent the infarct size at the acute phase of myocardial infarction; the lesion may either decrease in size during the healing process or increase due to extension. Recently, we investigated the relationship between infarct size estimated from total CK released and the site and severity of coronary lesions evaluated by selective coronary arteriography two months after the onset of infarction in 59 patients[18]. Our results showed that the site of the coronary lesion in the left anterior descending artery is the major determinant of infarct size; additionally, occlusion of the first diagonal branch results in a large infarction, while in disease of the right coronary artery, variations in the perfusion area of the right coronary artery in the posterior wall of the left ventricle are a major determinant of infarct size. Unlike the location of coronary lesions, the severity of coronary narrowing is unlikely to be related to infarct size.

4.4 CLINICAL LIMITATIONS IN ASSESSING INFARCT SIZE FROM TOTAL CK RELEASE

Sobel's method or the modified method of Norris et al. are widely used in coronary care units to assess infarct size by the serial determination of serum CK or CK-MB isoenzyme activities. Recently, however, some criticisms of this method have been raised. Roe et al. found that CK enzyme estimates lead to marked underestimates of the infarct size when the infarct is extremely large[19]. Cairns et al. also noticed that there is a substantial difference in CK enzyme estimates between homogeneous and scattered infarctions[20]. These criticisms are probably derived from the substantial difference between large and small infarcts in the washout rate of CK in the interstitial space from the infarcted myocardium. Rapid inactivation of CK activity in the cardiac lymphatics may also contribute to this discrepancy between the enzyme estimate and the histologically determined infarct size; the prolonged contact of CK with cardiac lymph during its slow transport from the center of a large homogeneous infarction might lead to extensive local destruction, as noted by Cairns et al.[20]

However, results reexamined by Swain et al. indicate that total CK released correlates well ($r=0.94$) with the histological extent of infarction in canine hearts when infarct weight is less than 20 g. However, over a large range of infarctions, the relationship between enzyme estimate and histologically determined infarct size is best described as being a power function rather than a linear function[21]. These reports suggest that Sobel's method may underestimate the size of an extremely large infarct. Contrary to this, another criticism raised is the possibility that total CK released may lead to an overestimation of infarct size when reperfusion occurred during the early phase of infarction. Vatner et al. found that total CK released was augmented with reperfusion after 1 or 4 h after coronary occlusion[22]. These results also suggest that regional myocardial blood flow may play an important role in washing the CK out into the circulation. Therefore, total CK released may be unable to provide an assessment of infarct size when regional myocardial blood flow is altered by angioplasty and thrombolytic therapy, for example.

Despite these limitations, serum CK activity is still widely used as a clinical index of infarct size, providing useful information.

REFERENCES

1. Wilkinson, J.H.: Clinical significance of enzyme activity measurements. *Clin. Chem.* 16: 882-890, 1970.
2. Inoue, M., Hori, M., Nishimoto, Y. et al.: Immunological determination of serum m-AST activity in patients with acute myocardial infarction. *Brit. Heart J.* 40: 1251-1256, 1978.
3. Spieckermann, P.G., Nordbeck, H. & Preusse, C.J.: From heart to plasma. In *Enzymes in Cardiology, Diagnosis and Research*, ed. by Hearse, D.J. and Deleiris, J. pp. 81-95, John Wiley & Sons, Chichester, N.Y., Brisbane, Toronto, 1979.
4. Posen, S.: Turnover of circulating enzymes. *Clin. Chem.* 16: 71-84, 1970.
5. Standjord, P.E., Thomas, K.E. & White, L.P.: Studies on isocitric and lactic dehydrogenases in experimental myocardial infarction. *J.Clin. Invest.* 38: 2111-2118, 1959.
6. Hori, M., Fukui, S., Nishimoto, Y. et al.: Disappearance rates of serum enzymes in acute myocardial infarction: Their relation to duration of elevated serum enzyme activities. *Med. J. Osaka Univ.* 25: 167-176, 1975.
7. Hori, M., Fukui, S., Nishimoto, Y. et al.: A method for the estimation of peak serum LDH activity based on the single post-peak level after acute myocardial infarction. *Jpn. Heart J.* 18: 202-213, 1979.
8. Sørensen, N.S.: Creatine phosphokinase in the diagnosis of myocardial infarction. *Acta Med. Scand.* 174: 725-734, 1963.
9. Kjekshus, J.K. & Sobel, B.E.: Depressed myocardial creatine phosphokinase activity following experimental myocardial infarction in rabbit. *Circ. Res.* 27: 403-414, 1970.
10. Maroko, P.R., Kjekshus, J.K. Sobel, B.E. et al.: Factors influencing infarct size following experimental coronary artery occlusions. *Circulation* 43: 67-82, 1971.
11. Shell, W.E., Kjekshus, J.K. & Sobel, B.E.: Quantitative assessment of the extent of myocardial infarction in the conscious dog by means of analysis of serial changes in serum creatine phosphokinase activity. *J.Clin. Invest.* 50: 2614-2625, 1971.
12. Norris, R.M., Whitlock, R.M.L., Barratt-Boyes, C. et al.: Clinical measurement of myocardial infarct size. Modification of a method for the estimation of total creatine phosphokinase release after myocardial infarction. *Circulation* 51: 614-620, 1975.
13. Sobel, B.E., Markham, J., Korlsberg, R.P. et al.: The nature of disappearance of creatine kinase from the circulation and its influence on enzymatic estimation of infarct size. *Circ. Res.* 41: 836-844, 1977.
14. Inoue, M., Hori, M., Fukui, S. et al.: Evaluation of evolution of myocardial infarction by serial determinations of serum creatine kinase activity. *Brit. Heart J.* 39: 485-492, 1977.

15. Inoue, M., Hori, M., Fukunami, M. et al.: Evaluation of precordial ST segment mapping as an index of infarct size in patients with acute myocardial infarction. *Brit. Heart J.* 42: 276-733, 1979.
16. Sobel, B.E., Bresnaban, G.F., Shell, W.E. et al.: Estimation of infarct size in man and its relation to prognosis. *Circulation* 46: 640-648, 1972.
17. Hori, M., Inoue, M., Fukui, S. et al.: Correlation of ejection fraction and infarct size estimated from the total CK released in patients with acute myocardial infarction. *Brit. Heart J.* 41: 433-440, 1979.
18. Hori, M., Inoue, M., Ohgitani, N. et al.: Site and severity of coronary narrowing and infarct size in man. *Brit. Heart J.* 44: 271-279, 1980.
19. Roe, C.R., Cobb, F.R., Starmer, C.F. et al.: The relationship between enzymatic and histologic estimates of the extent of myocardial infarction in conscious dogs with permanent coronary occlusion. *Circulation* 55: 438-449, 1977.
20. Cairns, J.A., Missirlis, E. & Fallen, E.L.: Myocardial infarction size from serial CPK: Variability of CPK serum entry ratio with size and model of infarction. *Circulation* 58:1143-1153, 1978.
21. Swain, J.L., Cobb, F.R., McHale, P.A. et al.: Nonlinear relationship between creatine kinase estimates and histologic extent of infarctions in conscious dogs; Effects of regional myocardial blood flow. *Circulation* 62: 1239-1247, 1980.
22. Vatner, S.F., Baig, J., Manders, W.T. et al.: Effects of coronary artery reperfusion on myocardial infarct size calculated from creatine kinase. *J. Clin. Invest.* 61: 1048-1056, 1978.

8
INTRARENAL HEMO- AND URODYNAMICS EXAMINED BY FUNCTIONAL IMAGES WITH I-131 HIPPURAN RENOSCINTIGRAPHY

Tsunehiko Nishimura and Kazufumi Kimura

1. INTRODUCTION

Since it was first introduced by Winter and Taplan[1,2], the radioactive renogram, using I-131 hippuran, has been developed to the point where it is now a reliable screening test of renal hemo- and urodynamics. Parameters such as renal blood flow and urinary excretion which express renal function have been obtained quantitatively by 3-compartment (blood, kidney and bladder) analysis[3,4]. Since the conventional (total) renogram is the summation of the temporal distribution of a tracer at a given time following injection, the information provided by regional renal function is lost in a single display of the renogram. We have attempted to construct the "functional image" of sequential hippuran renoscintigraphy, which represents a spatial parametric map indicating regional renal function in the kidney[5,6]. In the following, we present: (a) a method for constructing the functional image of the kidney, (b) the clinical application of functional images including compartmental analysis and (c) the detection of lesions in patients with various renal diseases.

2. SUBJECTS

In 67 patients with various renal diseases and in 10 healthy subjects, functional images were obtained by sequential renoscintigraphy. There were 16 patients with focal lesions in the kidney including renal cyst and tumor; 14 with obstructive uropathy including hydronephrosis; 14 with renal vascular changes including renovascular hypertension or renal infarction; and 23 patients with diffuse parenchymal damage including chronic glomerulonephritis or renal failure.

3. PROCEDURE FOR DYNAMIC STUDY AND DATA PROCESSING

An Anger camera connected to an on-line minicomputer system was used to process the data. A dynamic curve was extracted from each element of the digitalized image of the kidney, and pertinent parameters representing renal function were calculated and displayed as functional images.

The location of the kidney was identified using a Tc-99 m DMSA renal scintigram. For the dynamic study, 400 μCi of I-131 hippuran was rapidly injected as a bolus intravenously and sequential images (each for 20 sec) of the kidney were recorded for 20 min with an Anger camera.

Each sequential image was digitalized on a frame of 64×64 matrix and stored in a magnetic tape. Each dynamic curve was constructed from four neighboring elements after smoothing was performed for nine-element data boundering each other. By such processing, the dynamic curves became sufficiently smooth for the following analysis.

The next step is the calculation of pertinent parameters from each dynamic curve, which reflect renal function. The parametric maps showing the spatial distribution of calculated parameters were constructed. The functional image was displayed on a CRT in the form of a 64×64 matrix by the interpolation technique, after the intensity of the brightness by shadows was normalized by 10 levels of the gray scale.

4. CALCULATION OF PARAMETERS

The parameters calculated from a dynamic curve are as follows:
(A) T_{max}, C_{max}, UP and DOWN SLOPE were the parameters frequently used in the evaluation of the conventional renogram (Fig. 1).
1. C_{max}: the maximum counts
2. T_{max}: the time interval between injection and C_{max}
3. UP SLOPE: the slope just before T_{max}
4. DOWN SLOPE: the slope immediately after T_{max}

Parameters (3) and (4) are calculated by linear approximation using the least squares method.

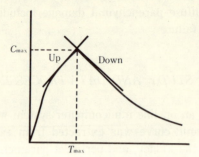

Fig. 1. Pertinent parameters chosen from the dynamic curve of each element are T_{max}, C_{max}, Up slope and Down slope.

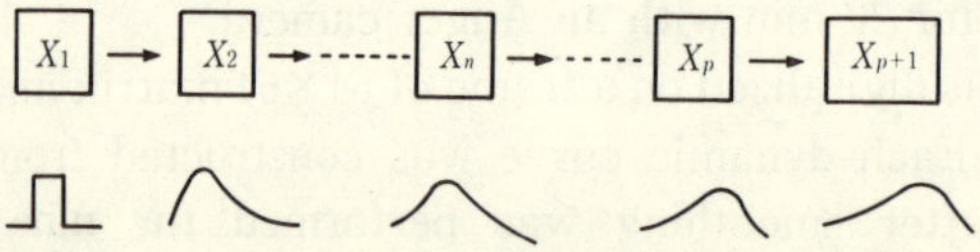

$$Q_n(T_n) = T_n \cdot X_n(T_n)/A_n \leq \frac{(n-1)^n}{(n-1)!}\exp(1-n)$$

- n : the minimum number of compartments which is the least value of n's satisfying the above inequality
- T_n : the time of the unique maximum of $X_n(T_n)$
- $X_n(T_n)$: the value of X_n at the maximum
- A_n : $A_n = \int X_n(t)\,dt$

Fig. 2. Determination of the number of precursor compartment from the dynamic curve of each element.

(B) Minimum numbers of precursor compartments in the dynamic curve were estimated using the method proposed by London and Hearon[7] (Fig. 2). In their method for a one-way compartmental model, i.e. $X_1 \to X_2 \to \cdots \to X_p \to X_{p+1}$, in which the tracer is initially given in compartment 1, the minimum number of precursor compartments is determined as follows: letting $Q_n(T)$ be $T_n X_n(T_n)/A_n$, where T_n is the time corresponding to the maximum of $X_n(t)$, $X_n(T_n)$, the maximum value of X_n, and $A_n = \int_0^\infty X_n(t)dt$, the minimum number of compartments is given by the least value n satisfying the inequality in Figure 2.

By applying this compartmental analysis for each dynamic curve, the number of compartments was calculated in each element of the kidney.

5. RESULTS AND DISCUSSIONS

Functional images were obtained in 67 patients with and 10 without renal disease. The results were evaluated clinically by comparing conventional renograms with radiographic procedures, such as intravenous pyelography and selective angiography.

The image of C_{max} is useful for assessing the total number of lesions, such as cysts and tumors of the kidney, where the count is relatively small compared with that of a normal area.

The image of T_{max} reflects transitional hemo- and urodynamics of the peak time of tracer in each element. Comparison of the regional dynamic curve with the total renogram shows that the tracer accumulated in the cortex and was excreted rapidly; in the pelvic area the intensity of radioactivity increased gradually. As a gradual time delay of T_{max} is observed from the cortex to the pelvis, the functional image of T_{max} agrees well with its anatomical structure when renal function is normal. On the other hand, T_{max} is significantly delayed in the lesion with ischemic and obstructive changes. The time delay of T_{max} is observed in the renal parenchyma, while that in the obstructive lesion may reflect urinary retention in the pelvic region.

The image of the UP SLOPE with a defective area corresponds to the focal lesions in renovascular changes, such as renovascular hypertension and renal infarction. Furthermore, the size of the ischemic area estimated by these procedures was in good agreement with angiographic findings.

The image of the DOWN SLOPE in the hydronephrotic portion is expressed as a defective area, while the remaining cortex with normal excretory function is clearly delineated from the impaired portion. The size and degree of hydronephrotic change are estimated from this functional image.

The images of precursor compartments revealed that the number of compartments is usually less than two in the cortex and five or six in the pelvic region when renal function is normal. The number of compartments does not correspond to the anatomical and physiological structure of the kidney but significantly represents the character of the dynamic curve. In

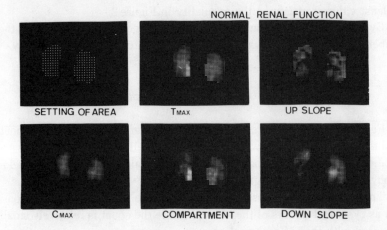

Fig. 3. Functional images in a normal subject. The image of T_{max} reflects the transitional changes of peak time in each element; a gradual increment is observed from cortex to pelvis. The individual images of compartments are similar to the image of T_{max}; the number of compartments is usually two in the cortex and five in the pelvic region. In the UP-SLOPE image, the cortex is seen in high density and the DOWN-SLOPE image reflects the excretory function of each element.

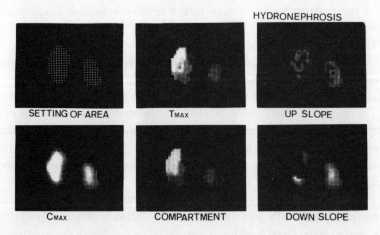

Fig. 4. Functional images in hydronephrosis. A significant time delay is observed in T_{max} and compartment images corresponding to an obstructive lesion caused by urinary retention. In the DOWN-SLOPE image, the lesion was expressed as a defect area.

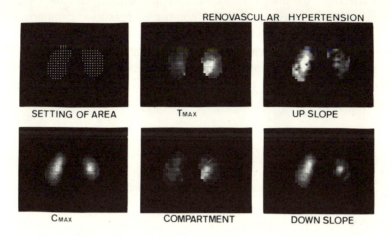

Fig. 5. Functional images in renovascular hypertension. A significant time delay is observed in T$_{max}$ and in compartment images corresponding to the ischemic lesion. In the UP-SLOPE image, the lesion was expressed as a defect area caused by stenosis of the renal artery.

Table. 1. Clinical significance of functional images of the kidney. In the five groups of renal diseases, each parametric map showed a characteristic image reflecting clinical significance.

	C$_{max}$	T$_{max}$	Number of compartments	Up slope	Down slope
Nomal renal function	peak count in central portion ↗ outer portion ↘	cortex→pelvis gradual delay	cortex : 2 pelvis : 5-6	cortex ↗ pelvis ↘	cortex→pelvis homogeneous
Obstructive uropathy	peak count in the lesion ↗	significant delay in the lesion	up to 8 in the lesion	unchanged cortex ↗ pelvis ↘	down slope ↘ defect in the lesion
Focal lesion	peak count in the lesion ↓	variable	variable	variable	variable
Renal vascular change	peak count in the lesion ↘	significant delay in the lesion	up to 8 in the lesion	up slope defect in the lesion	cortex→pelvis homogeneous
Renal parenchymal change	peak count in all areas ↓	cortex→pelvis longer delay homogeneous	cortex→pelvis homogeneous 3-6	cortex→pelvis homogeneous	cortex→pelvis gradual ↘

all cases studied, the images of the number of compartments were similar to those of T_{max}, indicating that the number of precursor compartments reflects delayed transport of tracer.

Some representative cases are shown in Figures 3, 4 and 5 and the clinical significance of parametric maps is summarized in Table 1. The functional images of these parameters proved to be useful for evaluating the regional distribution of kidney function.

6. CONCLUSION

1. The functional image obtained from serial hippuran renoscintigraphy was developed using an Anger camera connected to an on-line minicomputer.

2. The pertinent parameters extracted from the ordinary renogram were T_{max}, C_{max}, UP-and DOWN-SLOPE, and the number of precursor compartments. These five parameters, representing renal function, were displayed as functional images.

3. Renal functional images in patients with various renal diseases were useful for assessing the pathogenicity of the lesion and for detecting the lesion which would not otherwise be detected by conventional methods such as renography or scintigraphy. Findings from functional images agreed with those from the angiogram.

REFERENCES

1. Winter, C.C.: Clinical study of new renal function test; the radioactive diodrast renogram. *J. Urol.* 76 : 182-196, 1956.
2. Taplin, G.V., Meredith, O.M. et al.: The radioisotope renogram. *J. Lab. Clin. Med.* 48 : 886-901, 1956.
3. Coe, F.L. & Burke, G.: A theoretical approach to the I-131 hippuran renogram. *J. Nucl. Med.* 5 : 555-561, 1964.
4. Blaufox, M.D., Orvis, A.L., Owen, C.L. et al.: A compartment analysis of the radiorenogram and distribution of I-131 hippuran in the dogs. *Am. J. Physiol.* 204 : 1059-1064, 1963.
5. Kimura, K., Nishimura, T., Abe, H. et al.: A new method of analysis and display of intrarenal dynamics using functional images. In *Proceeding of Asian and Oceania Congress of Nuclear Medicine.* Sydney, Australia, 81-84, 1976.
6. Nishimura, T.: A new method of analysis and display of renal dynamics by functional images. *Jpn. J. Nucl. Med.* 14 : 105-121, 1977 (in Japanese).
7. London, W.P. & Hearon, T.Z.: Estimation of the number of precursors in a sequence of the first order reaction. *Math. Biosci.* 14 : 281-285, 1972.

9

AN ON-LINE MONITORING SYSTEM OF CEREBRAL BLOOD FLOW AND CEREBRAL OXYGEN CONSUMPTION

Yoshihiro Kuriyama

1. INTRODUCTION

Development of a day-by-day monitoring system for cerebral circulation and metabolism would make it possible to grasp the pathophysiology of acute cerebrovascular disease, to maintain adequate cerebral circulation during open heart surgery in high-risk patients with advanced cerebrovascular occlusion, and to control patients under barbiturate therapy to better understand barbiturate-induced changes in cerebral blood flow and metabolism. It would also help to decide therapeutic indications and estimate the efficacy of various kinds of therapy.

Currently, cerebral blood flow is commonly determined with radioactive tracers or N_2O. In monitoring cerebral circulation, the following basic conditions are necessary:

1. Blood samples need not be collected since determinations must be repeated more than several times a day.
2. Tracers should be available at reasonable prices.
3. Tracers should be nonradioactive, since determinations are made in intensive care units, operating rooms, and wards.
4. Tracers should be inert.

To satisfy the above conditions, we developed a system for determining cerebral blood flow, using argon gas and a medical mass spectrometer.

This chapter deals with the on-line data processing system and the results of cerebral blood flow and oxygen consumption determinations. The development of this system has made it possible to know the various indices of cerebral circulation and metabolism immediately after they are measured.

2. METHODS

2.1 ON-LINE DATA PROCESSING SYSTEM

The main components of the data processing system are two medical mass spectrometers (MEDSPECT II, Chemetron Co., USA), and a minicomputer (DEC-LAB 03, DEC Co., USA).

The block diagram of the on-line data processing system is shown in Figure 1. The outputs of the medical mass spectrometers are fed into the central monitor, which was available in the stroke care unit (SCU) to monitor such signs as arterial blood pressure and respiration.

Arterial blood pressure and respiration impedance curve signals, as well as the partial pressures of various gases in arterial and venous blood, determined by medical mass spectrometers, are all fed simultaneously into the computer from the central monitor. The sampling time is 0.5 sec.

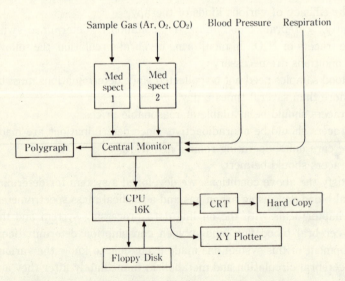

Fig. 1. Block diagram of the on-line data processing system.

2.2 DETERMINATION OF CEREBRAL BLOOD FLOW

The internal jugular vein was punctured by the introducing catheter, a 19-gauge, 15-cm long needle with a silicone sleeve, and the tip of the introducing catheter was inserted down into the internal jugular bulb where it was retained.

A special adaptor was connected to the introducing catheter, and a silastic catheter from the medical mass spectrometer was inserted through its opening and fixed so that the tip of the silastic catheter protruded about 2 cm from the tip of the introducing catheter. The special adaptor is designed to prevent blood from flowing back through the gap between the silastic catheter and the introducing catheter. Also, blood can be collected through another opening. A femoral artery was also punctured and the silastic catheter fixed in the same way with its tip properly protruding into the blood stream.

The patient then inhaled a mixture of argon : oxygen : nitrogen (1 : 1 : 3). Inhalation of this argon-containing gas was stopped when equilibrium was reached, and room air was then inhaled. The in vivo partial pressures of argon in the femoral artery and internal jugular vein were fed into the computer.

2.3 CALCULATION OF CEREBRAL BLOOD FLOW

Kety and Schmidt[1] measured cerebral blood flow based on Fick's principle. According to Henry's law, the calculation formula is expressed in terms of partial pressure from the desaturation curve.

$$CBF = P_v(T_s)\lambda / \int_0^{T_s} (P_v - P_a) dt \tag{1}$$

CBF : cerebral blood flow
P_v : partial pressure of argon in the venous blood
P_a : partial pressure of argon in the arterial blood
T_s : desaturation time
λ : brain-blood partition coefficient

In the restless patient with acute cerebrovascular disease, the following problems may arise at the time of the measurement.

1. Even if the argon gas mixture is inhaled sufficiently, variations in respiration may prevent the partial pressure of argon from stabilizing in arterial and venous blood.

2. Violent body movements may change the position of the silastic

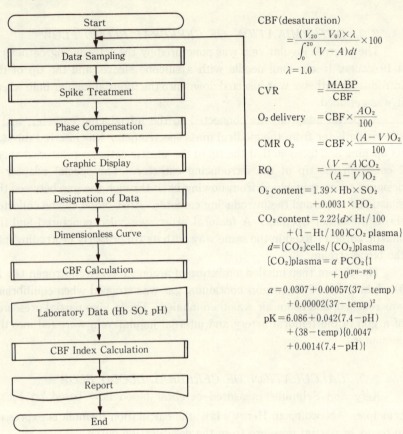

Fig. 2. Flow chart and calculation formula for cerebral circulation parameters.

catheter in the vascular lumen. To solve the above two problems, the argon desaturation curve obtained has been made dimensionless. That is, the starting points of the desaturation curves of arterial and venous blood have been set at 1 and the time of completion at 0. Equation 1 is modified as follows:

$$CBF = \lambda / \sum_{i=l}^{N} (X_{vi} - X_{ai}) \Delta t \qquad (2)$$

Δt : sampling time (0.5 sec)
N : Ts 60/0.5
X_{ai} : dimensionless value of arterial partial pressure of argon
X_{vi} : dimensionless value of venous partial pressure of argon

After cerebral blood flow, Hb, Hct, pH, SO_2 and body temperature are calculated, the values are fed from the keyboard and, in addition to the data measured on-line, values for cerebral circulation and metabolism are obtained from the calculation schema shown in Figure 2.

3. RESULTS

3.1 CBF CALCULATION AND X-Y PLOTTER OUTPUT

Figure 3 shows the dimensionless curve, as well as CBF, mean $PaCO_2$ at 20 min and average mean arterial blood pressure presented simultaneously on the X-Y plot.

3.2 OUTPUT TO HARD COPY

The cerebral blood flow and metabolism results are output from the CRT and hard copy, as shown in Figure 4. The data on the cerebral blood flow and metabolism were fed into the computer on line, and CBF, MAP (average mean arterial blood pressure for the 20 min of the desaturation process), APO_2 (arterial blood PO_2), $APCO_2$ (arterial blood PCO_2), VPO_2 (venous PO_2) and $VPCO_2$ (venous PCO_2) were computed. The laboratory data, such as Hb, Hct, PHA (arterial pH), PHV (venous pH), SAO_2 (arterial blood SO_2), SVO_2 (venous blood SO_2) and T (body temperature

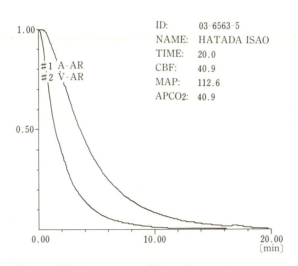

Fig. 3. X-Y plotter output of Argon desaturation curves.

```
*************** REPORT ***************
DATE : MARCH 13.198010:00          TIME : 10:00

ID    :03-6563-5              NAME  :HATADA ISAO
AGE   : 45                    WEIGHT:58.00
SEX   :M                      HEIGHT: 170.00
COMMENT:
RIND,R-CCA 55% STENOSIS, R-ICA 35% STENOSIS, PRE-O

**** ANALYSIS DATA ****
            FIRST         SECOND         THIRD
 CBF  :     40.9          42.6           0.0
 MAP  :     112.          108.           0.
 APO2 :     99.4          90.9           0.0
 APCO2:     40.9          40.2           0.0
 VPO2 :     40.5          39.0           0.0
 VPCO2:     51.6          50.9           0.0


**** LABORATORY DATA ****
            FIRST         SECOND         THIRD
 HB   :     11.800        11.800         0.000
 HT   :     39.500        39.500         0.000
 PHA  :     7.394         7.401          0.000
 PHV  :     7.336         7.343          0.000
 SAO2 :     98.700        97.900         0.000
 SVO2 :     57.200        54.800         0.000
 T    :     37.000        37.000         0.000

************** INDEX ******************
            FIRST         SECOND         THIRD
 CVR    :   2.7384        2.5352         0.0000

 (A-V)O2 :  6.9894        7.2301         0.0000

 O2 DEL2 :  6.7472        6.9606         0.0000

 CMRO2  :   2.8587        3.0800         0.0000

 (V-A)CO2:  5.7079        5.8072         0.0000

 RQ     :   0.8167        0.8156         0.0000
```

Fig. 4. Results of cerebral circulation parameters.

expressed in °C) were input from the keyboard. From these data, the indeces shown in Fig. 4 were calculated.

The indices include CVR (cerebral vascular resistance), $(A-V)O_2$ (arteriovenous oxygen difference), O_2DEL (oxygen delivery), $CMRO_2$ (cerebral metabolic rate of oxygen), $(V-A)CO_2$ (arteriovenous CO_2 content difference) and RQ (respiratory quotient). The above results are produced as a 15 cm×15 cm report, and attached to the medical record.

3.3 VALUES BY THE PRESENT METHOD
The following mean values were obtained in six subjects: cerebral

Table 1. Cerebral circulation parameters in control series

Case	Age	CBF	MAP	PaCO$_2$	CVR	CMRO$_2$	O$_2$-Delivery
1. Male	51	53.1	76	43.2	1.43	3.30	8.5
2. Male	32	58.7	86	41.8	1.47	4.04	11.3
3. Female	50	52.8	79	42.7	1.49	3.06	8.3
4. Male	47	50.1	97	43.0	1.94	3.96	10.1
5. Male	65	57.7	81	41.4	1.40	4.10	12.8
6. Male	35	64.0	99	38.6	1.54	4.32	12.1
Mean	46.7	56.1	86	41.8	1.55	3.80	10.5
±SD	±12.0	±5.1	±9.6	±1.7	±0.2	±0.5	±1.9

CBF (cerebral blood flow) : ml/100g/min, MAP (mean arterial pressure): mmHg, PaCO$_2$: mmHg,
CVR (cerebrovascular resistance) : mmHg/ml/100g/min,
CMRO$_2$ (cerebral metabolic rate of oxygen) : ml/100g/min, O$_2$-Delivery : ml/100g/min

blood flow, 56.1 ml/100 g/min; PaCO$_2$, 41.8 mmHg; and mean arterial pressure, 86 mmHg. The cerebral metabolic rate of oxygen was 3.80 ml/100 g/min, and cerebral vascular resistance 1.55 mmHg/ml/100 g/min (Table 1). The reproducibility of the cerebral blood flow by the present method, the ratio of the difference between the measured values in the first and second measurements to the value in the first, was 5.1±3.8%.

4. DISCUSSION AND CONCLUDING REMARKS

The *in vivo* determination of blood gas pressure using a medical mass spectrometer is designed to analyze gas through a special stainless steel, tube catheter with pores at its tip and coated with a silicon diffusion membrane[2,3]. This method has the following advantages: (a) it can continuously and simultaneously determine the partial pressure of oxygen, carbon dioxide and argon, and (b) it can maintain stability for determinations over a long period of time.

Values determined by this method are adequately reliable; they have been reported to correspond with those reported for the Radiometer method over a wide range, from high to low, of oxygen and carbon dioxide[3]. Good static properties were also seen for argon in our studies[4]. Hence, accuracy does not seem to be a problem in cerebral blood flow determinations.

The method requires a semipermeable membrane through which gas is collected. The catheter, with silicon membrane, is distined to yield lower values than one with a teflon membrane, if the flow rate is less than 4 cm/sec^2, since it consumes much more gas. Although this does not present problems in arterial determinations, further studies seem to be required for venous determinations. However, the flow rate in the human internal jugular vein, determined with a Doppler flowmeter, is 30-50 cm/sec[5] so that flow dependence should not cause errors in *in vivo* gas determinations for blood from the internal jugular vein.

The normal value for CBF by this method was 56.3±9.6 ml/100 g/min, which is close to that obtained using previous methods[1,6].

Pevsner[7], who used the present method in patients convalescing from head injuries, obtained an average of 50.8±5.3 ml/100 g/min. Linearity of the method was reported by Dyken[8], Hass et al.[9] and Ishikawa et al.[10] Dyken who compared cerebral blood flow determinations by the argon desaturation method with that by the Kr^{85} desaturation method, found that both methods were highly comparable, since the error of determination was just 7.2±5.7%. Hass et al. compared cerebral blood flow values determined by the N_2O and argon desaturation methods, and found that CBF by N_2O was equivalent to 1.13 CBF by argon. Ishikawa[10] reported that the mean ratio of direct CBF to argon CBF was 1.008±0.106 in animal experiments. These authors reported approximate values, suggesting that there are some problems with the linearity of the present method.

As for the brain-blood partition coefficient (λ), which becomes as issue in calculations of cerebral blood flow, Pevsner[7] employed 1.0 and Silver[11], 0.95. Ishikawa[10], who made 50 determinations in animals by the direct method, reported it was 0.96. Recently, Ohta et al.[12] measured the brain-blood partition coefficient of various inert gases, and noted that it was 1.077±0.029 for argon. However, it is questionable as to whether the brain-blood partition coefficient value of normal brain tissue, determined in vitro in animal experiments, may be applied to human brain tissue in various pathological conditions. Accordingly, the authors calculated cerebral blood flow by λ as 1.00.

The reproducibility of cerebral blood flow values by this method was 5.1±3.8%, which appeared to be fully comparable to the other method[13].

The present method for determining cerebral blood flow by measuring blood gas *in vivo*, using argon and a medical mass spectrometer, proved to be sufficiently linear, reproducible and accurate to compare favorably with other methods. It does not require blood collections and is free from the risks of exposure to radioactivity, so that we were able to determine cerebral circulation several times, before and during ST-MC bypass surgery, in a 2-year-old infant with "moya moya" disease.

It is hoped that this CBF monitoring system will be accepted as a useful instrument for studies of the pathophysiology of cerebrovascular disease, as frequent and repeated studies can be undertaken in a large number of cases at any time and place.

REFERENCES

1. Kety, S.S. & Schmidt, C.F.: The nitrous oxide method for the quantitative determination of cerebral blood flow in man: theory, procedure and normal value. *J.Clin. Invest.* 27: 476-483, 1948.
2. Brantigan, J.W., Gott, V.L., Vestal, M.L. et al.: A nonthrombogenic diffusion membrane for continuous in vivo measurement of blood gases by mass spectrometry. *J.Appl. Physiol.* 28: 375-377, 1970.
3. Brantigan, F.W., Dunn, K.L. & Albo, D.: A clinical catheter for continuous blood gas measurement by mass spectrometry. *J. Appl. Physiol.* 40: 443-446, 1976.
4. Kuriyama, Y., Sawada, T., Karasawa, J. et al.: Monitoring system of cerebral blood flow and cerebral metabolism. Part I. Measurement of cerebral blood flow and cerebral oxygen consumption by use of argon and mass spectrometry in clinical cases. *Respirat. Circ.* 29: 147-152, 1981, (in Japanese)
5. Nimura, Y., Kinoshita, N., Sakakibara, H. et al.: Blood flow measurement by the ultrasonic method. *Clin. Exam.* 22: 1449-1454, 1978, (in Japanese).
6. Lassen, N.A., Feinberg, I., & Lase, M.H: Bilateral studies of cerebral oxygen uptake in young and aged normal subjects and in patients with organic dementia. *J. Clin. Invest.* 38: 491-500, 1960.
7. Pevsner, P.H., Bhushan, C., Walker, A.E. et al.: Cerebral blood flow and oxygen consumption. An online technique. *Johns Hopkins Med. J.* 128: 134-140, 1971.
8. Dyken, M.L: Cerebral blood flow and metabolism studies comparing Krypton 85 desaturation technique with argon desaturation technique using the mass spectrometer. *Stroke* 3: 279-285, 1972.
9. Hass, W.K., Wald, A., Ransohoff, J. et al.: Argon and nitrous oxide cerebral blood flows simultaneously monitored by mass spectrometry in patients with head injury. *Eur. Neurol.* 8: 164-168, 1972.
10. Ishikawa, T., Nagai, K., Fukuda, S. et al.: Cerebral blood flow measurement by the mass spectrometer with argon—comparison with the direct method. *Clin. Physiol.* 7: 444-451, 1977-1979, (in Japanese).
11. Silver, D.J., Roberts, M., Owens, G. et al.: Measurement of regional blood flow. A comparison of the mass spectrographic and intra-arterial Xenon 133 techniques. *Neurology (Minneap.)* 24: 322-324, 1974.
12. Ohta, Y., Ar, A. & Farhi, I.E.: Solubility and partition coefficients for gases in rabbit brain and blood. *J.Appl. Physiol. Respirat. Environ. Exercise Physiol.* 46: 1169-1170, 1979.
13. Dyken, M.L., Campbell, R.L. & Frayser, R.: Cerebral blood flow, oxygen utilization and vascular reactivity: Internal carotid artery complete occlusion versus incomplete occlusion with infarction. *Neurology (Minneap.)* 20: 1127-1132, 1970.

10

THE TIME COURSE FOR THE DECLINE IN MINIATURE END-PLATE POTENTIAL FREQUENCY FOLLOWING TETANIC STIMULATION OF THE MOTOR NERVE

Hiroshi Kita, Kazuhiko Narita and William Van der Kloot

1. INTRODUCTION

After a motor nerve is stimulated tetanically in a Ca^{2+}-containing saline solution, the frequency of miniature end-plate potentials (min.e.p.p.s) increased, followed by a decline to the resting level [1-4]. A similar increase in the frequency of min.e.p.p.s occurs when neuromuscular preparations are exposed to an ionophore that can transport divalent cations, if the extracellular solution contains Ca^{2+} [5], or when the preparation is soaked in isotonic $CaCl_2$ [6]. Therefore, it is possible that the post-tetanic increase in the frequency of min.e.p.p.s is brought about by a rise in the concentration of Ca^{2+} ($[Ca^{2+}]$) at critical sites in the nerve terminal, and that the frequency declines as the Ca^{2+} is sequestered, relocated, or eliminated.

When Ca^{2+} is removed from the saline solution and replaced with Mg^{2+}, Co^{2+}, or Ni^{2+}, stimulation of the motor nerve no longer elicits the synchronous release of acetylcholine (ACh) [7-11]. However, tetanic stimulation in solutions prepared with these divalent metal cations (Mt^{2+}) in place of Ca^{2+} leads to a marked increase in the frequency of min.e.p.p.s. At the end of stimulation, the min.e.p.p. frequency slowly declines to the pre-stimulus level [12-16].

We interpret the sequence as follows: each time the nerve is stimulated, some of the Mt^{2+} enters the terminal. The increase in the intracellular $[Mt^{2+}]$ causes the rate of spontaneous release to increase. Whether the metals act directly in the terminal by mimicking the action of Ca^{2+} in the release sequence, or indirectly by causing the intracellular release of Ca^{2+}, is not known. We do know that a similar increase in the min.e.p.p. frequency occurs when the metals are transported into the terminal by the ionophores X-537A or A23187[5,17,18].

Based on compartmental analysis, the time course for the decline in min.e.p.p. frequency following tetanic stimulation was studied in saline solution containing Ca^{2+}, Mn^{2+}, Co^{2+}, or Ni^{2+}. The effects of temperature on the decline was determined as a probe for the mechanisms involved in decreasing the $[Mt^{2+}]$ within the terminal. The unusual metals, as well as Ca^{2+}, were studied because with them treatments to eliminate contraction can be avoided, which might be advantageous in further experiments. The major conclusion is that the decline in min.e.p.p. frequency under these circumstances has a low temperature sensitivity, in marked contrast to the high temperature sensitivity for the fall-off in the probability of quantal release following a nerve impulse in normal saline solution[19]. It seems likely that there is a two-stage mechanism for ending elevated quantal release following stimulation.

2. EFFECTS OF Ca^{2+} AND TEMPERATURE ON THE DECLINE IN MIN.E.P.P. FREQUENCY FOLLOWING A TETANUS

2.1 TIME COURSE FOR THE DECLINE AND ITS COMPARTMENTAL ANALYSIS

The experiments were performed on the sciatic nerve—sartorius muscle preparation from well-fed frogs (*Rana pipiens* or *R. temporaria*) or bullfrogs (*R. catesbeiana*). Min.e.p.p.s were recorded with an intracellular glass electrode using conventional equipment and techniques. The muscle chamber was surrounded by a jacket through which temperature-regulated water was circulated.

The bathing solution contained (mM) : NaCl, 100 ; KCl, 2.0 ; $CaCl_2$ (or in the experiments described in sections 3, 4 and 5 $MnCl_2$, $CoCl_2$, or $NiCl_2$), 2.5 ; and tris maleate buffer (pH 7.4), 8.0. The solutions also contained 10^{-6} g/ml neostigmine bromide. When the experiments were performed in 2.5 mM-Ca^{2+}-saline solution, muscles were pretreated with glycerol to eliminate contraction[20].

In each experiment a control sequence of min.e.p.p.s was first recorded on a chart recorder. Then, unless otherwise specified, the motor nerve was stimulated via a pair of silver electrodes for 2 min at 50 Hz with supramaximal shocks, 0.2 msec in duration. The number of min.e.p.p.s in each 15-, 30-, or 60-sec time bin was counted from the record.

The decline in the min.e.p.p. frequency after the tetanus appeared to follow a roughly exponential time course. To determine the parameters of the decline, we used a method devised by Provencher[21,22], in which the data are initially transformed to obtain good starting estimates for a non-linear least-squares analysis. The program fits the data with one to four exponentials, and calculates which of these gives the best fit:

$$\text{min.e.p.p. frequency} = F_\phi + \sum_{i=1}^{4} F_i \exp(-t/\tau_i),$$

where t is the time, τ_i the time constant, F_i the frequency at $t=0$ associated with the ith component of the decay, and F_ϕ the final, sustained min.e.p.p. frequency. A UNIVAC 1110 program fits the data. Average data are summarized as the mean value plus or minus the standard error of the mean value of several observations, the number of which is n.

2.2 EFFECTS OF Ca^{2+} AND TEMPERATURE ON THE DECLINE

Figure 1 shows an experiment with a sartorius muscle pretreated by the glycerol shock method to eliminate contractility. At 6.5°C, min.e.p.p.s were recorded. The broken line indicates the average frequency before tetanus. The motor nerve was then stimulated tetanically for 1 min, shown by the dark bar at the top. The min.e.p.p.s could not be counted during the

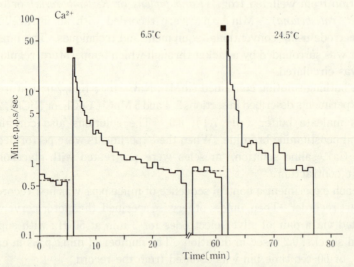

Fig. 1. An experiment in Ca^{2+}−saline solution.

tetanus because muscle action potentials developed. At the end of the stimulation, the min.e.p.p. frequency was 48 times the control level. The post-tetanic rise in the min.e.p.p. frequency was followed by a relatively rapid decline. Following recovery, the temperature was raised to 24.5°C and the same tetanus—recovery sequence was recorded. Again tetanus produced a substantial rise in min.e.p.p. frequency (73 times the pre-tetanus level), followed by a decline back to the resting level. Even a casual inspection of the records suggests that the rate of decline following the tetanus was not markedly slowed at low temperatures.

The data were quantified by fitting the best exponential to the decline (see 2. 1). At 24—27.5°C the mean time constant for the decline was 77±16 sec ($n=12$). At 5—8°C, the mean time constant was almost the same, 96 ±24 sec ($n=10$). The Q_{10}'s for the decay were calculated from paired experiments at single end-plates. The mean Q_{10} (from 5°C to 27.5°C) was 1.4±0.02 ($n=8$).

The method used to fit the decline in min.e.p.p. frequency fits the data points with one to four exponentials, and estimates the number of components that fit best. For the experiments in Ca^{2+}-saline solution at 5—8°C, a single exponential model gave the best fit in seven of the experiments; a double exponential model gave the best fit in the remaining three. At 24-27.5°C, the single exponential model fitted best in five experiments and the double exponential model fit the remaining seven. When a second exponential was detected, the second component had a slower time constant, ranging from 60 to 350 sec, and F_2 was 10 to 20 % of F_1.

Though the increase in min.e.p.p. frequency during the tetanus could not be measured in Ca^{2+}-saline solution because muscle action potentials developed, the mean Q_{10} (from 5°C to 26.5°C) for the ratio of the maximum frequency after stimulation for 1 min at 50 Hz to the pre-tetanus frequency was found to be 2.08±0.61 ($n=6$).

3. EFFECT OF Mn^{2+} AND TEMPERATURE ON THE DECAY CURVE

Figure 2A summarizes an experiment in Mn^{2+}-saline solution along with some of the original data (Fig. 2B). In Figure 2B, the upper records were obtained just before the first tetanus; the middle records, during the last 1.6 sec of the tetanus, and the lower records 10 min after the end of the tetanus at 8°C (left) and 20°C (right). During the tetanic stimulation of the

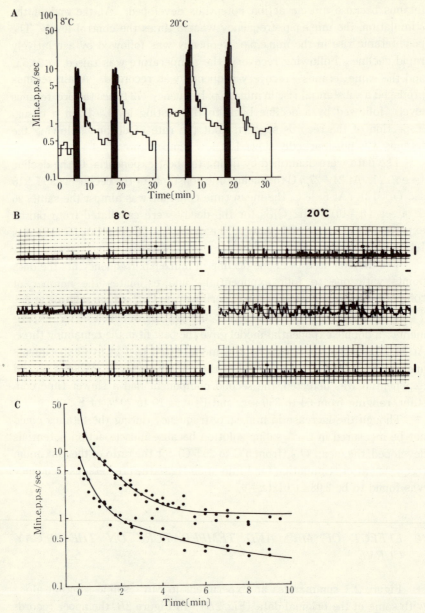

Fig. 2. A, an experiment in Mn^{2+}-saline solution. *B*, sample records of min.e.p.p.s obtained in Mn^{2+}-saline solution on which *A* is based. Calibrations: vertical, 1 mV; horizontal, 1 sec. *C*, the data from *Fig. 2A* plotted along with the curves calculated on the basis of a 2-component model.

nerve, no action potentials or end-plate potentials appeared. However, there was a notable rise in min.e.p.p. frequency during the stimulation (as shown by the dark bars in Fig. 2A), followed by a decline to the resting level. Similar behavior has previously been observed in Ca^{2+} free saline solutions containing Mg^{2+}, Co^{2+}, or Ni^{2+} [13,14]. The first point to notice in Figure 2A is the reproducibility of the results from trial to trial. Two stimulations were carried out at 8°C. In the first, the min.e.p.p. frequency increased 30-fold; in the second, it increased 29-fold. The time to recovery following tetanus is quite similar in all trials. At 20°C the frequency increased 26-fold after the first stimulation; in the second example, the increase was 29-fold.

Figure 2C shows the same data plotted along with the decay curve giving the best fit, as calculated by Provencher's method. The data best fit a 2-exponential model. Similarly, in three additional experiments in Mn^{2+}- saline solution, the data best fit a 2-exponential model. At 20—25°C, the time constants were 24 ± 9 sec ($n=8$) and 131 ± 28 sec ($n=8$). At 7—10°C, they were 24 ± 9 sec ($n=8$) and 201 ± 43 sec ($n=8$). The temperature sensitivity was calculated from experiments on individual muscles. The Q_{10} for the shorter time constant was 1.5 ± 0.4 ($n=5$), while that for the longer time constant was 1.2 ± 0.2 ($n=5$). As with the Ca^{2+}- saline solution, the decline in frequency following the tetanus has a low Q_{10}.

When the experiments are performed in Mn^{2+}-saline solution, min.e.p.p. frequency can be followed during the tetanus, since there is no phasic, stimulated release. From experiments on single end-plates at two different temperatures, the Q_{10} for the increase in min.e.p.p. frequency, produced by stimulation for 2 min at 50 Hz, is about 3.5 ± 0.9 ($n=5$).

4. EFFECTS OF Co^{2+} AND TEMPERATURE ON THE DECAY CURVE

An experiment in Co^{2+}-saline solution is illustrated as Figure 3. The tetanic stimulation (shown by the solid bars) at 7°C produced a tenfold increase in min.e.p.p. frequency. When stimulation ceased, the frequency was sustained at the elevated level for the next 45 min, which was as long as the observations continued. Since there was no recovery, the next part of the experiment was performed on the second preparation from the same frog, set up at 26°C. Now tetanic stimulation produced about a 51-fold increase in frequency; following the end of stimulation there was a decline

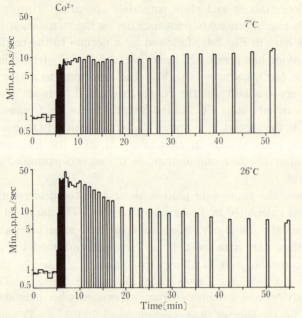

Fig. 3. An experiment in Co^{2+}-saline solution.

to what appears to be a steady, sustained plateau, with the frequency still at about 10 times the resting level. Similar results were obtained in two additional experiments. In each case the decay curves were best described by a 2-exponential curve with $\tau_1 = 25 \pm 10$ sec ($n=3$) and $\tau_2 = 296 \pm 30$ sec ($n=3$).

5. EFFECTS OF Ni^{2+} AND TEMPERATURE ON THE DECAY CURVE

The experiments at low temperature in Ni^{2+}-saline solution had quite a different outcome, as is shown in Figure 4. At 5°C the tetanus (solid bars) produced a 13-fold increase in min.e.p.p. frequency. After the end of stimulation there may have been a transitory decrease in min.e.p.p. frequency, but then there was a gradual rise to a sustained level equal to the highest frequency attained during the tetanus. The elevated frequency was sustained for more than 1 h after the tetanus. A similar sequence was observed in two other experiments.

Time Course of Min.e.p.p. Frequency after Tetanus

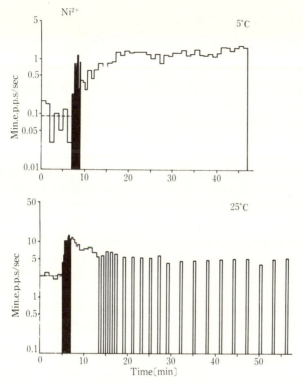

Fig. 4. An experiment in Ni^{2+}-saline solution.

Since there was no recovery from the effects of tetanic stimulation at low temperature, the second muscle from the same frog was used for the experiment at high temperature. An example is shown in Figure 4. When the muscle was at 25°C, tetanic stimulation caused a fivefold increase in min.e.p.p. frequency. After the tetanus was over, the frequency declined to a plateau that was about two times the control level. The plateau was sustained for almost 1 h after the tetanus, when observations ceased. The decay curve to the plateau was best fit by a 2-exponential model with $\tau_1 = 10$ sec and $\tau_2 = 46$ sec. Two additional experiments gave similar results.

6. TEMPERATURE AND Ca^{2+} SEQUESTRATION

We have studied two factors influencing the decline in min.e.p.p. frequency following tetanic stimulation of the motor nerve: (a) different extracellular divalent cations and, (b) different temperatures. When the nerve was stimulated repetitively in a solution containing 2.5 mM-Ca^{2+} or Mn^{2+} as the sole divalent cation, min.e.p.p. frequency rose substantially. After the tetanus ended, the frequency declined along an exponential or double exponential time course. The time constant for the decline in frequency appeared to be slightly dependent on temperature: the Q_{10} was about 1.4. When 2.5 mM-Co^{2+} or Ni^{2+} was the sole divalent cation, the min.e.p.p. frequency did not recover to the pretetanus level. The data can be interpreted as follows: assuming that the frequency of min.e.p.p.s depends on $[Ca^{2+}]$ at release activating sites in the motor nerve terminal, tetanic stimulation might increase $[Ca^{2+}]_{in}$ and thereby the frequency of min.e.p.p.s. The subsequent decline in min.e.p.p. frequency might reflect a decrease in $[Ca^{2+}]$ at these sites, caused by sequestration or transport. The rise in min.e.p.p. frequency in Mn^{2+} saline might occur because Mn^{2+} mimics the releasing action of Ca^{2+}, or it might release Ca^{2+} from intracellular storage sites.

The sustained increase in min.e.p.p. frequency following stimulation in Co^{2+} or Ni^{2+} could result from persistent binding of these divalent cations to critical sites near the release apparatus, or from a depressant effect on Ca^{2+} sequestration or transport.

Our findings on the effect of temperature on the decline in min.e.p.p. frequency following tetanic stimulation in Ca^{2+}-saline can be compared to those reported by Katz and Miledi[19], who determined the effects of temperature on the dispersion in time of quantal releases in the interval immediately after a nerve stimulation. We have taken the data from their Figure 7 and used it to calculate the fall-off in release probability, using the methods described in this paper. At 2.5°C and at 17.5°C the results best fit a 2-component model; at 7°C a single component model fits best. In each case, the single component model was used to calculate the Q_{10}'s. This system is markedly temperature sensitive: between 17.5°C and 7°C the Q_{10} is about 3.4. Between 17.5°C and 2.5°C the Q_{10} is about 8.6. Obviously there is a notable difference in the temperature sensitivity for the fall-off in release probability during the interval of enhanced quantal release immediately following nerve stimulation, and for the decline in min.e.p.p. frequency following a tetanus, although both are likely to reflect the decline in $[Ca^{2+}]$ at the release sites.

7. A TWO-STAGE MODEL FOR THE DECLINE

To account for the difference, we suggest that [Ca^{2+}] is reduced at release activating sites following nerve stimulation by a two-stage mechanism. Stage I operates at the relatively high Ca^{2+} levels that immediately follow stimulation, during which time several hundred quanta are normally released. This process has a high Q_{10}. Stage II is seen when the [Ca^{2+}] at the release sites is below the level needed for massive release; it operates more slowly than stage I to reduce [Ca^{2+}] to its resting level. This process has a low Q_{10}.

Several mechanisms have been suggested for removing Ca^{2+} from release sites in motor nerve terminals: diffusion, Na^+-Ca^{2+} exchange, sequestering in mitochondria or smooth endoplasmic reticulum. At least two of these mechanisms have a high Q_{10}. In the squid axon the Na^+-Ca^{2+} exchange system has a Q_{10} of about 3^{23}. Ca^{2+} sequestration by a preparation from rat brain synaptosomes (probably smooth endoplasmic reticulum) has a Q_{10} between 5°C and 30°C of about 3.0, and between 5°C and 12.5°C of about 5.8 [24,25]. This system is powered by ATP hydrolysis and can take up Ca^{2+} from levels as low as $0.3\mu M$.

Mitochondria take up divalent cations by two mechanisms, one involving ATP hydrolysis and the other based on the electrical negativity of the interior generated by the extrusion of protons[26,27]. Presumably the ATP-driven system has a relatively high Q_{10}. It is clear, therefore, that three mechanisms for removing Ca^{2+} are known to exist in nerves that have the temperature sensitivity required for our stage I.

Stage II has a relatively low Q_{10}. Several possibilities come to mind: diffusion, uptake into mitochondria, and a membrane exchange mechanism with a low Q_{10}.

As mentioned earlier, one uptake mechanism in mitochondria depends on internal electronegativity. As long as the proton gradient is maintained, this mechanism might have a low Q_{10}. The membrane Na^+-H^+ exchange mechanism in muscle sarcolemma has a low Q_{10} [28], so a low temperature sensitivity for such a system is not completely without precedent.

The final mechanism we thought of is diffusion. At first this would seem to be improbable as the time required is longer than 1 min, which is clearly far longer than the time required for the diffusion of Ca^{2+} from one point to another in a cross-section of nerve terminal. However, if Ca^{2+} enters close to release sites in the terminal, higher concentrations should be held in the Debye layer of the inner face of the axon than in the axoplasm. If Ca^{2+} is reversibly bound at many sites in the membrane, then the concentration near release sites might remain high for an appreciable period, as Ca^{2+} adheres to and leaves the binding sites until it diffuses to other parts of the terminal.

8. SUMMARY

When frog nerve-muscle preparations are stimulated tetanically in saline solutions containing Ca^{2+}, Mn^{2+}, Co^{2+}, or Ni^{2+}, min.e.p.p. frequency rises substantially. After stimulation is ended, the min.e.p.p. frequency decreases toward pre-stimulus levels. If we assume that min.e.p.p. frequencies are an index of the concentration of divalent cations at some critical site in the nerve terminal, the decline in min.e.p.p. frequency reflects the clearance of the divalent cation from the critical region. As a first step in investigating the clearing mechanism, we studied the effects of temperature on the decline in min.e.p.p. frequencies following a tetanus. The Q_{10}'s for the fall in min.e.p.p. frequencies following the tetanus in Ca^{2+} or Mn^{2+}, range between 1.2 and 1.6. The results can be interpreted in terms of a two-stage model for the fall-off in release probability following stimulation. In Co^{2+} or Ni^{2+} containing solutions at 7°C or lower, the min.e.p.p. frequency is sustained at an elevated level following the tetanus; at higher temperatures the decline does not reach the initial control level.

ACKNOWLEDGMENT

We are grateful to Elsevier/North-Holland Biomedical Press for permission to essentially reproduce our paper published in *Brain Research*, 190: 435-445, 1980.

REFERENCES

1 Braun, M., Schmidt, R.F. & Zimmermann, M.: Facilitation at the frog neuromuscular junction during and after repetitive stimulation. *Pflügers Arch. Ges. Physiol.* 287: 41-55, 1966.
2 Brooks, V.B.: An intracellular study of the action of repetitive nerve volleys and of

botulinum toxin on miniature end-plate potentials. *J. Physiol.* (*Lond.*) 134:264-277, 1956.
3   Hubbard, J.I.: Repetitive stimulation at the mammalian neuromuscular junction, and the mobilization of transmitter. *J. Physiol.* (*Lond.*) 169: 641-662, 1963.
4   Liley, A.W.; An investigation of spontaneous activity at the neuromuscular junction of the rat. *J. Physiol.* (*Lond.*) 132: 650-666, 1956.
5   Kita, H. & Van der Kloot, W.: Effects of the ionophore X-537A on acetylcholine release at the frog neuromuscular junction. *J. Physiol.* (*Lond.*) 259: 177-198, 1976.
6   Heuser, J., Katz, B. & Miledi, R.: Structural and functional changes of frog neuromuscular junctions in high calcium solutions. *Proc. Roy. Soc. B* 178: 407-415, 1971.
7   Balnave, R.J. & Gage, P.W.: The inhibitory effect of manganese on transmitter release at the neuromuscular junction of the toad. *Br. J. Pharmac.* 47: 339-352, 1973.
8   Jenkinson, D.H.: The nature of the antagonism between calcium and magnesium ions at the neuromuscular junction. *J. Physiol.* (*Lond.*) 138: 434-444, 1957.
9   Mambrini, J. & Benoit, P.R.: Action du nickel sur la libération du transmetteur à la jonction neuro-musculaire. *C. R. Séanc. Soc. Biol.* 161: 524-528, 1967.
10 Meiri, U. & Rahamimoff, R.: Neuromuscular transmission: inhibition by manganese ions. *Science* 176: 308-309, 1972.
11 Weakly, J.N.: The action of cobalt ions on neuromuscular transmission in the frog. *J. Physiol.* (*Lond.*) 234: 597-612, 1973.
12 Blioch, Z.L., Glagoleva, I.M., Liberman, E.A. et al.: A study of the mechanism of quantal transmitter release at a chemical synapse. *J. Physiol.* (*Lond.*) 199: 11-35, 1968.
13 Hurlbut, W.P., Longenecker, H.B., Jr. & Mauro, A.: Effects of calcium and magnesium on the frequency of miniature end-plate potentials during prolonged tetanization. *J. Physiol.* (*Lond.*) 219: 17-38, 1971.
14 Kita, H. & Van der Kloot, W.: Action of Co and Ni at the frog neuromuscular junction. *Nature New Biol.* 245: 52-53, 1973.
15 Miledi, R. & Thies, R.: Tetanic and post-tetanic rise in frequency of miniature end-plate potentials in low-calcium solutions. *J. Physiol.* (*Lond.*) 212: 245-257, 1971.
16 Silinsky, E.M., Mellow, A.M. & Phillips, T.E.: Conventional calcium channel mediates asynchronous acetylcholine release by motor nerve impulses. *Nature* (*Lond.*) 270: 528-530, 1977.
17 Kita, H., Madden, K. & Van der Kloot, W.: Effects of the "calcium ionophore" A-23187 on transmitter release at the frog neuromuscular junction. *Life Sci.* 17: 1837-1842, 1975.
18 Statham, H.E. & Duncan, C.J.: The action of ionophores at the frog neuromuscular junction. *Life Sci.* 17: 1401-1406, 1975.
19 Katz, B. & Miledi, R.: The effect of temperature on the synaptic delay at the neuromuscular junction, *J. Physiol.* (*Lond.*) 181: 656-670, 1965.
20 Eisenberg, R.S., Howell, J.N. & Vaughan, P.C.: The maintenance of resting potentials in glycerol-treated muscle fibers. *J. Physiol.* (*Lond.*) 215: 95-102, 1971.
21 Provencher, S.W.: A Fourier method for the analysis of exponential decay curves. *Biophys. J.* 16: 27-41, 1976.
22 Provencher, S.W.: An eigenfunction expansion method for the analysis of exponential decay curves. *J. Chem. Phys.* 64: 2772-2777, 1976.
23 Baker, P.F.: Transport and metabolism of calcium ions in nerve. *Prog. Biophys. Mol. Biol.* 24: 177-223, 1972.
24 Blaustein, M.P., Ratzlaff, R.W., Kendrick, N.C. et al.: Calcium buffering in presynaptic nerve terminals. I. Evidence for involvement of a nonmitochondrial ATP-dependent sequestration mechanism. *J. Gen. Physiol.* 72: 15-41, 1978.
25 Blaustein, M.P., Ratzlaff, R.W. & Schweitzer, E.S.: Calcium buffering in presynaptic nerve terminals. II. Kinetic properties of the nonmitochondrial Ca sequestration mechanism. *J.*

Gen. Physiol. 72 : 43-66, 1978.
26 Lehninger, A.L. : Mitochondria and calcium ion transport. *Biochem. J.* 119 : 129-138, 1970.
27 Rottenberg, H. & Scarpa, A. : Calcium uptake and membrane potential in mitochondria. *Biochemistry* 13 : 4811-4817, 1974.
28 Aickin, C.C. & Thomas, R.C. : An investigation of the ionic mechanism of intracellular pH regulation in mouse soleus muscle fibres. *J. Physiol. (Lond.)* 273 : 295-316, 1977.

11

COMPARTMENTAL ANALYSIS IN PULMONARY PHYSIOLOGY, WITH SPECIAL REFERENCE TO THE DISTRIBUTION FUNCTION

Takao Ōkubo

Since the Fowler et al.'s report[1], compartmental analysis has been used by many investigators of respiratory physiology as a tool for analyzing uneven distribution of ventilation in the lungs, and has become a common technique for pulmonary function tests. On the other hand, the continuity in the degree of pathological change in diseased lungs suggests that they might be treated as a model with many compartments with different ventilatory characteristics. In 1962, Gomez et al.[2] and our group[3-7] independently introduced such techniques to describe uneven ventilation as a continuing distribution, using a distribution function. There is a great advantage in using the continuous distribution model rather than conventional 2-compartment models for describing pulmonary function. Over the past 20 years, such analysis has been extended to include the assessment of many gas exchange functions, i.e., ventilation, diffusion and pulmonary blood flow as well as mechanical functions of the lung.

1. DEFINITION AND DESCRIPTION OF UNEVEN DISTRIBUTION IN PULMONARY PHYSIOLOGY

Uneven distribution describes the state in which some material or phenomenon is distributed unevenly. To clarify this vague expression, I will use the example of beans spread out on a table (Fig. 1). Lines divide the table into nine square sections of the same size. Thus, uneven distribution can be seen by comparing the number of beans in each of the nine sections. Obviously, the distribution between sections *a* and *b* is uneven.

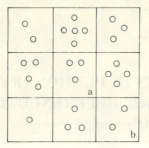

Fig. 1. A model of distribution where beans are spread on a table.

Even if the area of section *b* is increased until the number of beans equals that in *a*, the distribution of beans between the two sections is still not the same. Therefore, when we use the words even or uneven, we tacitly accept the concept of the number of beans (N) per unit area (A), i.e., N/A. The idea of N/A (i.e., a pair of parameters of two different phenomena) always appears when one tries to describe the distribution of some phenomenon. With the help of this concept, the distribution can be described quantitatively.

To describe the distribution of beans on the table in Figure 1, we have taken the number of beans in one unit (N/A) as the abscissa and the number of the section that has the same N/A as the ordinate. This gives a histogram (Fig. 2). As N/A is the key-word used to express distribution, we will call N/A a parameter of distribution. The ordinate expresses the amount of distribution (i.e., in this case the number of the section corre-

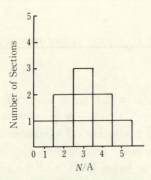

Fig. 2. A histogram expresses the distribution of beans on a table.

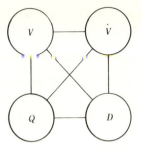

Fig. 3. Parameters of distribution in gas exchange are obtained by combination of two basic gas exchange parameters (V, $\dot{V}$, $\dot{Q}$ and D).

sponding to each value of N/A). The function that defines the relationship between the parameter and amount of distribution is called distribution function.

Regarding the nature of the parameter of distribution (A/B), we noticed that uneven distribution is a mismatch of phenomenon A and phenomenon B. Our concern is the kinds of mismatches that are evaluated when a gas exchange disturbance in the lungs is described. There are four functional values related to pulmonary gas exchange, i.e. lung volume (V), ventilation ($\dot{V}$), diffusion (D), and pulmonary blood flow ($\dot{Q}$). As illustrated in Figure 3, distribution parameters are a combination of these four basic values. Thus, there are six parameters of distribution for pulmonary gas exchange: $V/\dot{V}$, $\dot{V}/\dot{Q}$, D/V, $D/\dot{V}$, $D/\dot{Q}$ and $\dot{Q}/V$.

To clarify the meaning of distribution parameters for the measurement of functional unevenness, diffusing capacity will be discussed as an example. To assess the distribution of D/V, $D/\dot{V}$ or $D/\dot{Q}$ in the lung, different principles are used to measure diffusing capacity. To measure D/V, the single-breath method must be used to evaluate diffusing capacity; $D/\dot{V}$ distribution must be analyzed by the steady state method and $D/\dot{Q}$ by D_{O_2}, analyzing the concentration of oxygen in blood. Therefore, the principles of measurement are closely related to distribution parameters but not to the basic functional parameters. When the distribution of the distribution parameter in gas exchange function is evaluated, distribution corresponding to the ordinate in Figure 2 can be expressed in several ways. For example, in evaluating $V/\dot{V}$ distribution,[6,7] the distribution of ventilation having different $V/\dot{V}$ ratios, the distribution of lung volume concerning $V/\dot{V}$, and even the blood flow distribution corresponding to different $V/\dot{V}$ ratios must be considered. Such measures to quantify the amount of distribution are determined by selecting the sampling site for measurement, the principle for which is already selected corresponding to a given distribution parameter. For example, the distribution of $V/\dot{V}$ is analyzed by the multi-breath lung nitrogen washout test, wherein the ventilation distribution of $V/\dot{V}$ is determined by analyzing the nitrogen concentration of each breath at mouth level; lung volume distribution is analyzed by evaluating the total amount of expired nitrogen; and blood flow distribution is analyzed by determining the concentration of nitrogen in arterial blood during nitrogen washout.

2. DESCRIPTION OF THE DISTRIBUTION OF WASHOUT TIME CONSTANT[3,4,6]

Since Fowler et al.[1] reported their study, washout of a less soluble inert gas (e.g. nitrogen) in the lung has become widely used for the evaluation of uneven ventilation in the lungs. Breath-to-breath changes in the nitrogen concentration of expired air are evaluated by this technique after inspired gas is changed from air to pure oxygen. The concentration of nitrogen in expired air decreases with every breath (Fig. 4).

The washout from the simplest model——an alveolar-bronchial system with a single washout characteristic, i.e., homogenous lung (Fig. 5)——

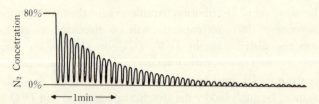

Fig. 4. An example of decrease in endotidal N_2 concentration in lung N_2 washout.

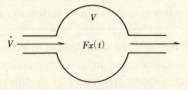

Fig. 5. A model for the analysis of N_2 washout from a single lung unit.

—will be described. In this figure, inspiratory and expiratory pathways have been separated and ventilation with a constant flow rate considered. V represents lung volume, $\dot{V}$ is ventilation, and $F_{N_2}(t)$ is the concentration of nitrogen in the lung after t minutes from the beginning of the washout. $V \cdot F_{N_2}(t)$ represents the amount of nitrogen in the lung at time t; the rate at which the quantity of nitrogen in the lung decreases is expressed by $dV \cdot F(t)/dt$, which is equal to the amount of nitrogen carried out the lung through ventilation. Therefore, the following equation is derived:

$$\frac{dV \cdot F_{N_2}(t)}{dt} = -F_{N_2}(t) \cdot \dot{V}.$$

Solving this differential equation and adding the concentration of nitrogen during air breathing, $F_{N_2}(0)$, to the equation as an initial condition gives:

$$F_{N_2}(t) = F_{N_2}(0) e^{-\frac{t}{T}},$$

where $T = V/\dot{V}$. T is the washout time constant or the time required for the initial alveolar nitrogen concentration to decrease to the value of $1/e$ of $F(0)$. Therefore, the smaller the value of T, the faster the nitrogen is washed out of the lungs, and vice versa.

If the washout time constants are unevenly distributed within the lung, and the lung consists of two compartments with time constants T_1 and T_2, the nitrogen concentration in expired air at time t is expressed as:

$$F_{N_2}(t) = \frac{\dot{V}_1 \cdot F_1(t) + \dot{V}_2 \cdot F_2(t)}{\dot{V}}$$

$$= \frac{\dot{V}_1}{\dot{V}} F_{N_2}(0) e^{-\frac{t}{T_1}} + \frac{\dot{V}_2}{\dot{V}} F_{N_2}(0) e^{-\frac{t}{T_2}},$$

where $\dot{V}_1$ and $\dot{V}_2$ are ventilations, and $F_1(t)$ and $F_2(t)$ are nitrogen concentrations in compartments I and II after t minutes of washout.

In a lung composed of n compartments, nitrogen concentration in mixed expired air is expressed as:

$$F_{N_2}(t) = \frac{F_0}{\dot{V}} \sum_{i=1}^{n} \dot{V}_i \cdot e^{-\frac{t}{T_i}}.$$

Setting $n \to \infty$, since the lung is composed of a very large number of compartments, and substituting $\dot{V}_i$ by the term $\dot{V}(T_i) dT$, this equation can be rewritten as follows:

$$F_{N_2}(t) = \lim_{n \to \infty} \frac{F_0}{\dot{V}} \sum_{i=1}^{n} \dot{V}(T_i) dT \cdot e^{-\frac{t}{T_i}}$$

$$= \frac{F_0}{\dot{V}} \int_0^\infty \dot{V}(T) e^{-\frac{t}{T}} dT, \qquad (1)$$

where $\dot{V}(T)$ is defined as

$$\dot{V}_E = \int_0^\infty \dot{V}(T) dT,$$

in which $\dot{V}_E$ is the total ventilation and $\dot{V}(T)$ is the distribution of pulmonary ventilation as a function of the washout time constant.

Similar treatment is applied to the volume distribution of washout time constants. The amount of nitrogen $M_{N_2}(t)$ in mMol remaining in the lung during multi-breath washout is expressed as follows in the homogeneous lung:

$$M_{N_2}(t) = V_0 e^{-\frac{t}{T}},$$

where $V_0 = V \cdot F(0)$ and $M_{N_2}(t) = V \cdot F_{N_2}(t)$. For a lung composed of n compartments, the amount of nitrogen remaining in the lung is written as:

$$M_{N_2}(t) = \sum_{i=1}^{n} V_i(0) e^{-\frac{t}{T_i}},$$

in which $V_i(0)$ is the amount of nitrogen contained in the ith compartment, having washout time constant T_i, at the beginning of washout. Again, using the continuous distribution model for the treatment of data in lung N_2 washout, and by setting $V_i(0) = V(T_i) dT$, $M_{N_2}(t)$ becomes:

$$M_{N_2}(t) = \int_0^\infty V(T) e^{-\frac{t}{T}} dT, \qquad (2)$$

because the amount of nitrogen remaining in the lung at time t is the sum of the nitrogen in each compartment at time t. $V(T)$ in Eq. 2 is defined as

$$FRC \times F_0 = \int_0^\infty V(T) dT,$$

and $V(T)/F_0$ is the distribution of lung volume having time constant T.

The relationship between the distribution function $V(T)$ and N_2 washout curve $M(t)$ is shown in Figure 6, where the X, Y and Z axes represent washout time constants, time for washout, and amount of nitrogen in the lung, respectively. Since F_0 is almost equal in each compartment throughout the lung, lung volume distribution with respect to washout time

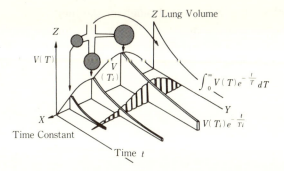

Fig. 6. A model explaining the relationship between distribution function of lung volume $V(T)$ and lung nitrogen washout curve $M(t)$. (For explanation, see text)

constants is shown on the X-Z plane, representing the continuous distribution of lung volume corresponding to the wide range of washout time constants from zero to infinity. The nitrogen washout curves from these compartments are shown three-dimensionally as exponential decreases from each initial nitrogen volume in the direction of time, parallel to the Y axis. The summation of washout curves for each compartment constitutes the total lung N_2 washout curve, illustrated on the Y-Z plane. As can be easily understood from the figure, the lung N_2 washout curve $M(t)$ is related to the distribution function $V(T)$ by some definite mathematical relationship, i.e., Laplace transform.[6] Therefore, once $V(T)$ is determined, nitrogen elimination $M(t)$ from the lung can be estimated. When $M(t)$ is observed in a wide range of washout times, the continuous distribution of lung volume $V(T)$ can be calculated as a function of washout time constant.

3. DESCRIPTION OF THE DISTRIBUTION OF MECHANICAL TIME CONSTANT IN THE LUNG[5]

When force is applied to the lung, ventilation is determined by the mechanical properties of the lung, which are usually analyzed using a model with singular viscoelastic behavior. However, the lung is really composed of a large number of parallel units, each with its own mechanical time constant (compliance × resistance). Therefore, an approach similar to that used in the nitrogen washout curve could be applied to the analysis of the distribution of mechanical time constants throughout the lung.

Regarding the lung as a single model consisting of a volume-elastic unit with a compliance C and a flow-resistive unit with a resistance R in series, the total pressure across the system at any moment is expressed as :

$$P = \frac{V}{C} + R\dot{V}.$$

When such a system is subjected to sinusoidal varying pressure,

$$P = P_0 e^{j\omega t}, \qquad (3)$$

the volume change in the model is expressed as follows:

$$V = V^* e^{j\omega t}, \quad V^* = CP_0 \frac{1}{1+j\omega T}, \quad T = RC, \qquad (4)$$

where P_0 is half the amplitude of the pressure swing. Thus, the complex compliance is given by Eqs. 3 and 4:

$$C^* = \frac{V}{P} = C\frac{1}{1+j\omega T} = C\frac{1}{1+\omega^2 T^2} - jC\frac{\omega T}{1+\omega^2 T^2}.$$

In the multi-compartmental model arranged in parallel, this equation is modified as follows:

$$C^* = \sum_{i=1}^{n} C_i \frac{1}{1+\omega^2 T_i^2} - j\sum_{i=1}^{n} C_i \frac{\omega T_i}{1+\omega^2 T_i^2}, \qquad (5)$$

where C_i and T_i are the compliance and the time constant of ith compartment. Introducing the distribution function with regard to the mechanical time constant——defined as $\int_0^\infty bF(T)dT = \lim_{n\to\infty}\sum_{i=1}^{n} C_i$——into Eq. 5, the complex compliance is conclusively expressed in the following equation:

$$C^* = b\int_0^\infty F(T)\frac{1}{1+\omega^2 T^2}dT - jb\int_0^\infty F(T)\frac{\omega T}{1+\omega^2 T^2}dT$$

or

$$Cd^* = b\int_0^\infty F(T)\frac{1}{1+\omega^2 T^2}dT, \qquad (6)$$

where Cd^* is that part of the complex compliance in phase with pressure.

4. DESCRIPTION OF THE DISTRIBUTION OF VENTILATION-TO-PERFUSION RATIO IN THE LUNG

The exchange of inert gas between the alveolar air and alveolar capillary blood reflects the ventilation-to-perfusion relationship ($\dot{V}/\dot{Q}$) in a unit of the lung; the magnitude of the exchange is related to the solubility of the inert gas. This phenomenon was initially introduced to assess the unevenness of $\dot{V}/\dot{Q}$ in the lung by Rochester et al.[8] and Farhi and Yokoyama[9], and applied to the analysis of continuous distribution of $\dot{V}/\dot{Q}$ in the lung by West and Wagner.[10,11]

In a homogeneous lung, inert gas exchange is described by Fick's equation (Fig. 7), wherein inert gas dissolved in saline is continuously infused into the mixed venous blood. When a steady state of inert gas exchange is achieved between inflow and outflow of inert gas in the lung unit, the following equation describes the inert gas exchange in the unit:

$$\dot{Q}_c \times C_{\bar{v}} = \dot{Q}_c \times C_a + \dot{V}_A \times F_A , \qquad (7)$$

where $\dot{Q}_c$, $\dot{V}_A$, C_a, $C_{\bar{v}}$, and F_A are the pulmonary blood flow, alveolar ventilation, inert gas contents in arterial and in mixed venous blood, and the concentration of inert gas in alveolar air, respectively. Since the inert gas is assumed to reach equilibrium between alveolar air and capillary blood, the content of the inert gas in both alveoli and capillary are partitioned according to Henry's law:

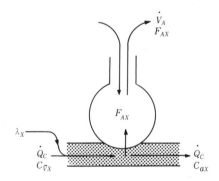

Fig. 7. A model showing the exchange of inert gas between pulmonary capillary and alveolus in a single lung unit.

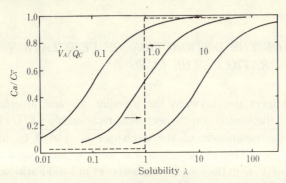

Fig. 8. The relationship between retention ratio $C_a/C_{\bar{v}}$ and solubility of inert gases λ for three different $\dot{V}/\dot{Q}$ values (0.1, 1.0 and 10). The curves for $\dot{V}/\dot{Q}=1.0$ could be simulated by the broken line when expansion of λ covers a very wide range.

$$C_a = \lambda \cdot F_A, \qquad (8)$$

where λ is the partition coefficient. The combination of Eqs. 7 and 8 introduces the following equation:

$$\frac{C_a}{C_{\bar{v}}} = \frac{1}{1+\frac{\dot{V}}{\dot{Q}} \cdot \frac{1}{\lambda}}. \qquad (9)$$

The term $C_a/C_{\bar{v}}$, called retention ratio, expresses the retention of inert gas in the blood following gas exchange in the lung.

In Figure 8, the relationship between $C_a/C_{\bar{v}}$ and λ in Eq. 9 is shown for three different $\dot{V}/\dot{Q}$ values (0.1, 1.0 and 10). A simple observation of the curve allows us to simulate each curve as a step function, the value of which changes from zero to one at the point of $\lambda = \dot{V}/\dot{Q}$, where the curve covers a very wide range of solubility. By applying this characteristic to many inert gases, the distribution of the $\dot{V}/\dot{Q}$ ratio can be obtained. An example is given in Figure 9, where the behavior of a compartment model with three different $\dot{V}/\dot{Q}$ ratios (upper panel) is presented for retention ratios with changes of λ (middle panel), and for the distribution pattern of $\dot{V}/\dot{Q}$ (lower panel), resulting from the analysis of retention ratio. The step-wise increase in the retention ratio with λ is shown in the middle panel. Blood flow distribution, as a function of the $\dot{V}/\dot{Q}$ ratio, is obtained as illustrated in the lower panel, where it is analyzed by differentiating retention ratio data by λ, the first approximation for the analysis of distribution function with these kinds of basic functions.

In the continuous distribution model, $C_a/C_{\bar{v}}$ could be described as

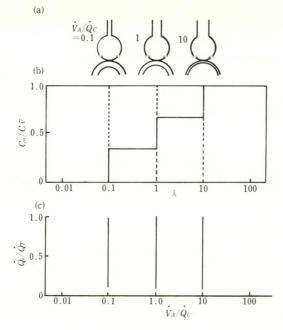

Fig. 9. A schematic representation of the analysis of $\dot{V}/\dot{Q}$ distribution using $C_a/C_{\bar{v}} - \lambda$ relationship. (a) Model of $\dot{V}/\dot{Q}$ distribution with three different $\dot{V}/\dot{Q}$ values (0.1, 1.0 and 10) perfused with the same amount of blood flow. (b) Changes in retention ratio with changes in the solubility of inert gases; where $C_a/C_{\bar{v}} - \lambda$ relationship is simulated as in Figure 8. (c) Blood flow distribution as a function of the $\dot{V}/\dot{Q}$ ratio obtained by the analysis of the $C_a/C_{\bar{v}}$ curve of Figure 9-b.

follows, by weighting the retention of inert gas of each compartment with its blood flows:

$$\frac{C_a}{C_{\bar{v}}} = \lim_{n \to \infty} \frac{1}{\dot{Q}} \sum_{i=1}^{n} \dot{Q}(\dot{V}/\dot{Q}_i) \frac{d\dot{V}/\dot{Q}}{1+(\dot{V}/\dot{Q})_i \cdot \frac{1}{\lambda}}$$

$$= \frac{1}{\dot{Q}} \int_0^\infty \dot{Q}(\dot{V}/\dot{Q}) \frac{d\dot{V}/\dot{Q}}{1+\dot{V}/\dot{Q} \cdot \frac{1}{\lambda}}. \tag{10}$$

The equation is similar to that for complex compliance in Eq. 6, where $\dot{V}/\dot{Q}$ and $1/\lambda$ correspond to ω^2 and T^2, respectively. Consequently, it is possible to use a similar method of analysis to obtain the continuous distribution of these parameters in the lung.

5. PATTERNS OF DISTRIBUTION FUNCTION IN NORMAL AND DISEASED LUNG

Distribution function is obtained by the mathematical inversion of the observed experimental curve described by Eqs. 1 and 2 for nitrogen washout,[4,6] Eq. 6 for complex compliance,[5] and Eq. 10 for the retention ratio of inert gases[10], respectively. Distribution functions obtained in this way are illustrated in Figures 10, 11, and 12.

In Figure 10, the frequency distribution curves of lung volume as a function of washout time constant are drawn as a dotted line for the normal subject (Fig. 10a) ; for those with chronic pulmonary emphysema (Fig. 10b), distribution of ventilation is drawn as a broken line.[6] In normal subjects, the peak of the volume distribution curve is symmetrical and sharp, with a relatively narrow range, the highest frequency is between 0.35 and 0.55 min.

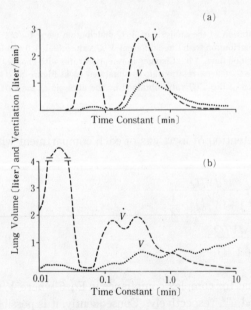

Fig. 10. Distribution of lung volume (V) and pulmonary ventilation ($\dot{V}$) concerning the washout time constant obtained by the lung N_2 washout in a normal subject (10-a) and in a patient with type A chronic obstructive lung disease (10-b). [From Ōkubo and Lenfant (6); reprinted by permission of the publisher]

This peak makes up most of the lung volume. There is a small volume peak for extremely short time constants between 0.04 and 0.08 min. The volume of this small peak is about 140 ml, suggesting a contribution by anatomical dead space. A typical pattern of volume distribution in diseased subjects is characterized by a very broad distribution of washout time constants and the absence of a definite peak (Fig. 10b, dotted line); a gradual ascending slope toward the long time constant without a decrease in frequency, suggests the highest frequency lies beyond the observed range of time constants. Again a small peak precedes the bulk of volume distributions. Two sharp peaks of ventilation distribution, seen in normal subjects, coincide with the peaks of lung volume curves. A high frequency component of ventilation distribution corresponds to the bulk of the lung volume distribution. However, this peak is always to the left (smaller time constant) of the highest peak of the lung volume distribution. There is also a high frequency distribution peak corresponding to the lowest peak of the lung volume distribution. In diseased subjects, the largest portion of ventilation was observed between 0.1 and 1.0 min. This corresponded to the relatively small fraction of lung volume characterized by a range of time constants identical to those for most of the lung volume in normal subjects. Only a negligible amount of ventilation corresponded to the bulk of the lung volume in the range of larger time constants. As a consequence, depending on its blood flow, the lung portion with normal time constants must have an extremely high signficance in terms of gas exchange. The highest frequency distribution

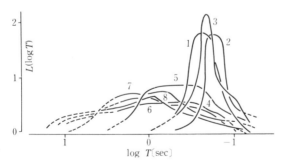

Fig. 11. Distribution of mechanical time constants obtained in healthy subjects (cases 1-3) and in patients with chronic pulmonary emphysema (cases 4-8). The abscissa and ordinate express time constant and its compliance, respectively. [From Nakamura et al. (5); reprinted by permission of the publisher]

resembling a peak of dead space ventilation found in normal subject was also observed.

The distribution of compliance as a function of the mechanical time constant is shown for normal individuals and for patients with chronic obstructive emphysema[5] in Figure 11. The curve in normal subjects peaks maximally in 0.2 sec, at which time it is narrow and roughly symmetrical with respect to the time constant. In contrast, a common feature of the distribution in emphysematous patients is a flat or trapezoidlike function distributed roughly between 0.1 and 10 sec, with a maximum peak at a much higher time constant than that of normal subjects. There is some resemblance between this distribution pattern of the mechanical time constant and the volume distribution of the washout time constant. This resemblance is understandable because the mechanical time constant partially

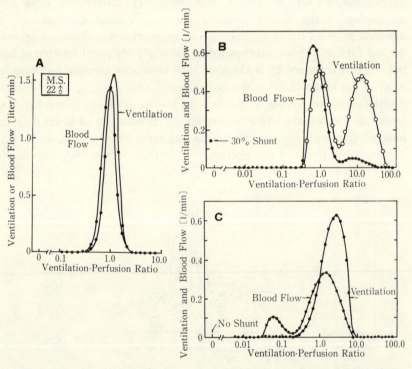

Fig. 12. Examples of distributions of ventilation-perfusion ratios in a normal subject and in patients with chronic obstructive lung disease. (A) The result from a young normal subject. (B) Typical distribution in a patient with type A COLD. (C) Distribution found in a patient with type B COLD. [From West[11]; reprinted by permission of the publisher.]

contributes to the value of the washout time constant.

With the permission of Dr. West, the distribution of his ventilation-to-perfusion ratio ($\dot{V}/\dot{Q}$) is shown in Figure 12.[11] Ventilation and blood flow were plotted on the ordinate against $\dot{V}/\dot{Q}$ on the abscissa in a logarithmic scale. The abscissa is broken to illustrate a compartment with a $\dot{V}/\dot{Q}$ of zero, i.e., "shunt." In Figure 12a, the distribution of ventilation and blood flow in a normal subject shows a narrow and skewed peak, spanning only one decade; there is no shunt.

Examples of $\dot{V}/\dot{Q}$ distribution in two patients with chronic pulmonary obstructive lung disease are shown in Figure 12b and c. Figure 12b shows typical patterns in patients with type A chronic obstructive lung disease (COLD). The patterns are bimodal and show a large amount of ventilation going to units with a high $\dot{V}/\dot{Q}$ ratio ($\doteqdot 3 \sim 80$), but less blood flow to these units. There is almost no blood flow to units with a $\dot{V}/\dot{Q}$ ratio below 0.3, and there is only a small shunt. The large amount of ventilation in high $\dot{V}/\dot{Q}$ units can presumably be explained as the result of parenchymal destruction in which the capillary bed is grossly decreased. By our observations,[6,7] these units are presumed to correspond to those with larger $V/\dot{V}$ values (slow space), as shown in Figure 10b. The distribution of $\dot{V}/\dot{Q}$ obtained from a patient with type B COLD is shown in Figure 12c. In a remarkable contrast to that of COLD type A, the blood flow to lung units with low $\dot{V}/\dot{Q}$ units between 0.02 and 0.1 is substantial, which may explain the more severe hypoxemia in patients with type B COLD.

As stated earlier, the distribution function is of great value because it specifically detects uneven pulmonary functions, especially in the pathological lung. It is widely applicable in many fields and accurately describes pulmonary functions mathematically. Examples of its applicability are its use for comparisons of physiological distribution data with anatomical distribution, the evaluation of respiratory physiology models by a more accurate description of distribution, and so on.

REFERENCES

1 Fowler, W.S., Cornish, E.R. Jr., & Kety, S.S.: Lung function studies. VIII. Analysis of alveolar ventilation by pulmonary N_2 clearance curves. *J. Clin. Invest.* 31: 40-50, 1951.

2 Goméz, D.M., Briscoe, W. & Cumming, G.: Continuous distribution of specific tidal volume throughout the lung. *J. Appl. Physiol.* 19: 683-692, 1964.

3 Ōkubo, T.: Pulmonary function tests in patients with chronic bronchitis (in Japanese). *Nippon Kyobushikkangakkai Zasshi* (JJTD) 2: 93-94, 1964.

4 Nakamura, T., Takishima, T., Ōkubo, T. et al.: Distribution function of the clearance time constant in lungs. *J. Appl. Physiol.* 21: 227-232, 1966.
5 Nakamura, T., Takishima, T., Sagi, Y. et al.: A new method of analyzing the distribution of mechanical time constants in the lungs. *J. Appl. Physiol.* 21: 265-270, 1966.
6 Ōkubo, T. & Lenfant, C.: Distribution function of lung volume and ventilation determined by lung N_2 washout. *J. Appl. Physiol.* 24: 658-667, 1968.
7 Lenfant, C. & Ōkubo, T.: Distribution function of pulmonary blood flow and ventilation-perfusion ratio in man. *J. Appl. Physiol.* 24: 668-677, 1968.
8 Rochester, D.F., Brown, R.A., Jr., Wichern, W.A. Jr. et al.: Comparison of alveolar and arterial concentrations of ^{85}Kr and ^{133}Xe infused intravenously in man. *J. Appl. Physiol.* 22: 423-430, 1967.
9 Farhi, L.E. & Yokoyama, T.: Effects of ventilation-perfusion inequality on elimination of inert gases. *Respir. Physiol.* 3: 12-20, 1967.
10 Wagner, P.D., Saltzman, H.A. & West, J.B.: Measurement of continuous distributions of ventilation-perfusion ratios: theory. *J. Appl. Physiol.* 36: 588-599, 1974.
11 West, J.B.: Ventilation-perfusion relationships (state of the art). *Am. Rev. Respir. Dis.* 116: 919-943, 1977.

12
APPLICATION OF KINETIC APPROACHES TO WATER AND ELECTROLYTE METABOLISM

Masahito Nagasaka

1. INTRODUCTION

Modeling in the compartmental analysis of water and electrolyte metabolism follows its practical purpose; the needed precision is a medical and clinical requirement. Direct analysis provides the most exact information about body composition, but a noninvasive technique, based on kinetic principles is more useful and dynamic pictures can often be obtained. One such study was the monumental compilation: The Body Cell Mass and Its Supporting Environments, by F.D. Moore, et al., published in 1963.[1] In the following, I discuss some achievements and restrictions in the analysis of water and electrolyte metabolism.

2. ONE-COMPARTMENT MODEL

A one-compartment approach is used to determine the pool size and turnover in a single or whole-body compartment. The turnover or metabolism of water and cations is distinguished by the fact that water is lost or acquired metabolically in the body space, whereas cations are unchanged. In general, water occupies a larger fraction and exchanges faster in the bodies of neonates and infants, but is slightly decreased in proportion and turnover in the elderly. This finding is particularly important in pediatric practice because diarrhea and vomiting readily cause dehydration in children. In a disease such as diabetes insipidus, the turnover rate of water increases considerably.

The turnover rate for sodium (Na) is a function of dietary intake[2].

However, it has been reported that the sodium space fluctuates unpredictably as though multiple gates were opening and closing at random to transfer the ion from many small compartments to a common pool[3].

Although a one-compartment model is simple, it does present some problems. First, equal distribution throughout the space is questionable. It is possible for a substance to be sequestered in some inactivating, irreversible compartment such as bone, where turnover is extremely slow, compared to the life span of the tracer in the body. Generally speaking, tracer mixing may not be guaranteed. The pool of tracer in bone is usually ignored in the clinical setting; total exchangeable amounts of tracer are sufficiently meaningful for many purposes. Second, although it is easy to calculate the balance, extrapolation with multiple sampling is required if a precise value is needed. Third, radioactive tracers pose a safety problem. For example, heavy water in a concentrated state may interfere with the body's chemical reactions and vital processes, and tritium may attach to genetic material. Finally, isotopes of hydrogen undergo molecular exchange with other constituent compounds in the body, although during the actual period of measurement the percentage is estimated to be only 1-2%[4].

3. RED BLOOD CELLS AND OTHER ISOLATED CELLS

Erythrocytes are easy to manipulate in vitro, and could possibly be treated as a simple one-compartment model. Close scrutiny, however, has revealed complexities and problems in modeling them, as well as other isolated cells, as a single compartment system. In theory, water may exist in red blood cells both in the free and in the non-solvent states. With the use of isotopically labeled water, this distinction is unnecessary.

Net cation flux is the difference between two oppositely directed unidirectional fluxes: cellular influx and efflux. Each unidirectional flux is subdivided into active, passive, carrier-mediated and facilitated transports, as well as exchange diffusion. Passive diffusion is sometimes called a leak. Active transport may be coupled to form a counter-transport or cotransport. In other cases an active transport will energize other seemingly active processes to form secondary active transport. Such transport systems often cannot reach a steady-state when the environment is changing, especially in the asymmetrically transporting epithelia, oscillatory excitable cells, and so on. In these cells one cannot expect physicochemical equilibrium as long as the cells live and work.

In kinetic terms, red blood cell Na shows free and bound or fast and slow fractions *in vitro*[5,6]. However, this may represent heterogeneity in the cell population. The size and density of pores or channels for a variety of ions and molecules can be estimated, and in a large cell the intracellular mobilities of these ions and molecules can be explored to define more precisely the components that are bound. Recently, studies with ion-selective intracellular electrodes for various anions and cations revealed that the activities in intracellular fluid may not be extrapolated from extracellular data. Clearly, further studies on intracellular physico-chemical states of water and electrolytes are needed.

4. 2-COMPATMENT MODEL

Heavy water is mixed fairly rapidly in the extracellular space. However, it has long been recognized that the cellular plasma membrane offers a small, but definite resistance to the diffusion of water. This resistance is greater than that to the penetration through an epithelial or cellular barrier. Plasma specific concentrations may be higher before they reach their final values. This inevitably calls for a 2-compartment model in kinetic analysis.

In isolated systems, relatively homogeneous tissue, such as skeletal muscle, cardiac muscle, and slices of brain or liver are thought to be composed of only 2-compartments——the intracellular and the extracellular spaces. This premise is generally fulfilled so long as one uses sufficiently small pieces of tissue in which diffusion in and out occurs almost instantaneously. However, problems arise when more than 3-compartments appear, particularly when the number of compartments in a tissue or organ differs between in vitro and in vivo conditions.

5. 3-COMPARTMENT MODEL

As discussed in the theoretical section, the 3-compartment model is the highest order of complexity that can be reached, if only the blood compartment is accessible for sampling. However, historically it was the model that fits the distribution of body fluids based on data from available tracers. That is,

total body water (TBW),

intracellular fluid (ICF),
extracellular fluid (ECF),
interstitial fluid (ISF), and
plasma volume (PV)

represent the anatomical compartments. They are determined by injecting tracers into the blood stream, which then diffuse into the extracellular space and from there into the total body water pool. Precise analysis of the dilution curves shows that the spaces obtained are not simply superimposed on the anatomical ones. The extracellular compartment is especially difficult to determine. First, its value differs according to the marker used, and it is often necessary to refer to the inulin space, sodium space, rhodan space, and so on. Second, at times the calculated spaces do not correspond to the anatomical structures. For example, the PV expands with time[7], and the ISF divides into two subspaces[8]. The former may be explained either by leakage of the marker protein molecules from the capillaries into the interstitial space, or by the circulation of plasma proteins outside the capillaries[9]. Also, the two ISF subspaces may represent the gel and free phases of the interstitial space[10,11]. However, even today it is difficult to allocate the spaces obtained to distinct anatomical structures.

These difficulties may be classified into several categories: (a) The first is the effective barrier function of compartment interfaces. The capillary wall is not a perfect semipermeable membrane and according to its location, its permeability to protein varies widely. The plasma membrane of the cell is generally permeable to water, but it has various channels and pumps for cations and anions and also has limited permeabilities to organic compounds used as tracers. Membranes comprised of epithelial cells have transcellular and intercellular permeabilities, and the latter may be tight or leaky. These cellular membranes may outline fluid cavities, such as the cerebrospinal fluid space and the articular and ocular sacs. Pathologically, ascites and pleural effusion would also make spaces. Channels and pathways often have selectivities, and cellular membranes may have pinocytosis and vesicular transport. (b) Disease states such as congestive heart failure, nephrotic syndrome, and cirrhosis of the liver with ascites may alter exchange kinetics profoundly and a steady-state sometimes cannot be expected. (c) If anatomical correspondence cannot be achieved, it is difficult to determine whether the model is in series or parallel, and intentional omission of any compartment will diminish the precision significantly.

6. MULTI-COMPARTMENT MODEL

This model is physiologically predetermined for calcium, magnesium, iron and other ions. However, Wilde remarked that even sodium or potassium may sometimes be multi-compartmentalized. He wondered whether these compartments represent organ systems or tissue fractions[12]. A probable distribution of compartment parameters among the tissues will also simulate a multi-compartment model.

7. SYSTEM DYNAMICS MODEL AND OTHER TOPICS

A complex model requires the help of a computer. Such complexity may arise when a regulatory model has control loops within it, or involves non-linearities. The kinetics and dynamics of regulatory agents are usually described by Michaelis-Menten type reactions, and this inevitably introduces non-linearity. If binding of such agents with receptors is included in the model, the apparent distribution volume expands and far exceeds the supposed anatomical space[13,14]. This experience has led investigators to adopt such expressions as nodes and loops rather than squares and arrows in compartmental analysis. It may be said allegorically that the concrete vision of fertile countries with touching borders is reduced to discrete oases with interconnecting caravans in a desert land.

Efforts have been made to simplify non-linear situations by employing quasi-linearization or by building a labyrinthine block to confine the non-linearities to a small region. However, the application of compartmental analysis to cellular transport processes has caused problems. The conventional electric circuit model sometimes can be translated into the compartmental model with some success; the evenly distributed parameter model can be treated similarly. The description of transport phenomena by Kedem-Katchalsky equations originally involves non-linearity. Linearization of these equations may again compete with compartmental analysis, which must be tested to determine its usefulness in such microscopic phenomena.

REFERENCES

1. Moore, F.D., Olesen, K.H., McMurrey, J.D. et al.: *The Body Cell Mass and Its Supporting Environment. Body Composition in Health and Disease.* Saunders, Philadelphia, 1963.
2. Threefoot, S., Burch, G. & Reaser, P.: The biologic decay periods of sodium in normal man, in patients with congestive heart failure, and in patients with the nephrotic syndrome as determined by Na^{22} as the tracer. *J. Lab. Clin. Med.* 34: 1-13, 1949.
3. Threefoot, S.A., Burch, G.E. & Ray, C.T.: Chloride "space" and total exchanging chloride in man measured with long-life radiochloride, Cl^{36}. *J. Lab. Clin. Med.* 42: 16-33, 1953.
4. Pinson, E.A.: Water exchanges and barriers as studied by the use of hydrogen isotopes. *Physiol. Rev.* 32: 123-134, 1952.
5. Gold, G.L. & Solomon, A.K.: The transport of sodium into human erythrocytes in vivo. *J. Gen. Physiol.* 38: 389-404, 1955.
6. Harris, E.J. & Prankerd, T.A.J.: Diffusion and permeation of cations in human and dog erythrocytes. *J. Gen. Physiol.* 41: 197-218, 1957.
7. Sapirstein, L.: Macromolecular exchanges in capillaries. In Reynolds, S.R.M. and Zweifach, B.W. (eds.): *The Microcirculation,* Univ. Ill. Pr., Urbana, 47-59, 1959.
8. Black, D.A.K.: *Essentials of Fluid Balance.* 4th ed. Blackwell, Oxford, 1967.
9. Casley-Smith, J.R.: The functioning and interrelationships of blood capillaries and lymphatics. *Experientia* 32: 1-12, 1976.
10. Wiederhielm, C.A.: Dynamics of transcapillary fluid exchange. in Chinard, F.P., Brooks, C.M., Dreizen, P. et al. (eds.): *Biological Interfaces: Flows and Exchanges,* Little, Brown, Boston, 29-61, 1968.
11. Brace, R.A.: Progress toward resolving the controversy of positive vs. negative interstitial fluid pressure. *Circ. Res.* 49: 281-297, 1981.
12. Wilde, W.S.: Transport through biological membranes. *Ann. Rev. Physiol.* 17: 17-36, 1955.
13. Gibaldi, M. & McNamara, P.J.: Apparent volumes of distribution and drug binding to plasma proteins and tissues. *Eur. J. Clin. Pharmacol.* 13: 373-378, 1978.
14. Gibalidi, M. & Koup, J.R.: Pharmacokinetic concepts-drug binding, apparent volume of distribution and clearance. *Eur. J. Clin. Pharmacol.* 20: 299-305, 1981.

13

APPLICATION OF COMPARTMENTAL MODEL OF SPLEEN HEMODYNAMICS TO *IN VIVO* EVALUATION OF RED CELL RHEOLOGY AND ITS DESTRUCTION

Yutaka Takahashi and Chikao Uyama

1. INTRODUCTION

The human spleen is a highly vascular organ of hemopoiesis and blood filtering[1]. Because of its recognition and its retention of even slightly defective cells which may escape entrapment by other filters, i.e., reticuloendothelial organs, it is considered the most sensitive and most refined filtering organ. The spleen's unique capability may be attributed to the circulation mode of blood cells. Concerning red cell rheology, the spleen is assumed to have the most complex features among body organs. Several dynamics studies have disclosed that cells are trapped in the microcirculation of this organ before they are actually lysed[2-5] and their rheology changes before the trapping[3-5]. These characteristic hemodynamic features, which require anatomic substantiation by further investigation of the fine structure of the vasculature[1,6,7], may reveal another functional aspect. A model of spleen hemodynamics is presented for the *in vivo* measurement and analysis of splenic hemodynamics and function. The model was used, in this study, to examine splenic rheology related to red cell destruction.

2. THE CHARACTERISTIC FEATURES OF SPLENIC HEMODYNAMICS AS A BASIS FOR A DYNAMICS MODEL

The following features of splenic hemodynamics were the basis of our model for in vivo measurements and the analysis of the results.

1. Because the arterial vessels terminate in different places and the connecting routes to the venous system are loose and variable[1], there are different and multiple pathways in the splenic microcircula-

tion.

2. Because of the redistribution of blood elements and plasma skimming in the distal portion of arterioles[3,6-8], plasma and cell elements may circulate separately.

3. There is a fast and a slow mode of red cell circulation that occur simultaneously: the faster has a circuit time comparable to that of plasma; the slower has a considerably retarded circuit time compared to plasma.

4. As a critical site in flow control, there is an anatomic restriction to the flow of red blood cells as they pass through slits in the sinus walls[8].

Based on these conceptual foundations, methods of experimental and clinical studies of spleen hemodynamics were selected, and kinetic models for simulation and for data analysis were designed.

3. DETERMINATION OF THE CHARACTERISTICS OF SPLEEN HEMODYNAMICS

3.1 A PERFUSION EXPERIMENT IN A DOG SPLEEN

To clarify the characteristics of the circulation through the spleen, an experiment was set up with isolated dog spleens. The splenic artery and vein were cannulated, and the spleen was then perfused with Ringer's solution at a certain flow rate by connecting the arterial cannula to a roller pump. Radiotracers were injected in a bolus through the arterial cannula. Radiograms of the 'input', 'output' and 'spleen' were obtained with scintillation detectors set over the arterial and venous cannula and the spleen.

First, a mixture of ^{99m}Tc albumin (^{99m}Tc-HSA) and ^{51}Cr red cells (^{51}Cr-RBC) was injected at different flow rates. Radiograms, corresponding to each tracer, were obtained with a pulse-height analyzer. Second, a mixture of technetium-albumin and radiogold, ^{198}Au, was injected by relatively slow perfusion; the 'spleen' and 'output' radiograms for each tracer were obtained and subjected to analysis.

The 'output' radiograms are shown in Figure 1 (left). The passage values for ^{99m}Tc albumin and ^{51}Cr red cells were plotted on the logarithmic scale. Two phases can be readily seen; the first or 'rapid phase' in which the tracer reaches a peak and then decreases rapidly, and the second or 'slow phase' in which the residues of tracer gradually exit from the spleen in the form of a tail. These rapid and slow phases of dynamics are clearly distinguishable in the ^{51}Cr red cell radiogram, compared to the plasma

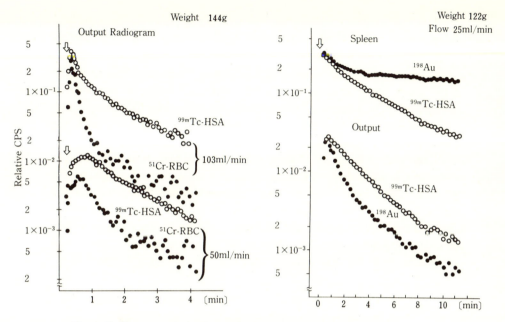

Fig. 1. Radiogram analysis of the isolated dog spleen under perfusion.

radiogram. Analysis of the 'output' radiogram revealed that the character of passage through the spleen is closely approximated by the sum of two exponential components, which correspond to the fast and slow dynamics phases. The peak-shaped dynamics of the rapid phase become distinct as flow rate increases but become obscure and diminish as flow rate decreases.

The results of the second experiment are shown in Figure 1 (right). The 'spleen' radiograms show that approximately 35% of the administered radiogolds were extracted and retained in the spleen, while all of the technetium-albumin flowed out. In the 'output' radiograms, the gold-colloid radiogram is steeper than the albumin radiogram, with a 65% greater rate of decline. These findings imply that extraction of the colloids took place in competition with their outflow, in other words, in the mode of the first order system which is subordinate to the flowing compartment(s). The interrelationship of 'input', 'output' and 'spleen' radiograms suggested that impulse-response analysis can be applied to the analysis of the radiosplenogram.

3.2 ANALYSIS OF RADIOGRAMS OF THE SPLENIC HILUS AND PERIPHERY

Using a scintillation camera, radiograms of the area of interest (AOI) of the spleen were obtained in an adult patient following an intraarterial injection of ^{99m}Tc albumin. Two radiograms were selected for analysis: one corresponding to the hilus (curve 1 and 2 in Fig. 2), and the other to the splenic periphery (curve 4).

Simulation was accomplished using a simplified model: τ_a and τ_v represent transport delays in the artery and vein, $1/(Ts+1)$ represents the first order delay in the capillary bed; different weights (w_1, w_2 and w_3) were given to different compartments (artery, capillary, and vein) for the hilus and periphery (upper right of Fig. 2). These findings indicated that the characteristics of the circulation in the spleen could be represented by a combination of the first order system and the appropriate time delay.

4. CLINICAL STUDIES: IN VIVO MEASUREMENT AND ANALYSIS OF SPLENIC HEMODYNAMICS

4.1 METHOD

The cases studied were divided into four groups: (a) control; (b) hereditary spherocytosis (HS), a hemolytic anemia caused by an intracor-

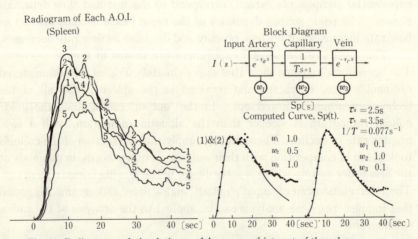

Fig. 2. Radiogram and circulation model on area of interest of the spleen.

puscular defect; (c) autoimmune hemolytic anemia, and (d) congestive splenomegaly with portal hypertension (CS), a splenic hypersequestration of red cells by an extracorpuscular factor. Hemodynamics of normal cells in HS spleen, those of HS cells in normal spleen, and spleen hemodynamics after porta-systemic shunting in patients with congestive splenomegaly were also studied.

In these studies ^{131}I- or ^{99m}Tc-HSA was used as the radiotracer in studies of plasma flow, and ^{51}Cr-labeled erythrocytes in studies of red cell flow.

Based on findings from previous experiments[3,5,11], three splenic compartments, each with different red cell flow dynamics——X-1, the fast path; X-2, the intermediate pool; and X-3, the slow pool——were postulated. There were two steps in the experiment: one for fast-phase dynamics with a transit time of 10 to 100 seconds, and the other for the slow phase with a transit time of 0.5 to more than 30 minutes.

4.1.1 Study of the Slow-Phase Dynamics

In the study of slow-phase dynamics, tracers were injected into the patient's antecubital vein, and radiograms of the spleen, precordium, and liver were obtained with collimated 1.5-inch NaI detectors. Blood samples were collected at appropriate time intervals to plot a blood dilution curve for the tracer. The curve was then supplemented and extrapolated to correspond to the radiosplenogram.

For analysis[12], X-1 was included in the systemic compartment, X-0 and two splenic pool compartments, X-2 and X-3, were set in parallel to X-0; 3-compartmental analysis was then applied (Fig. 3, right; Fig. 6).

4.1.2 Fast-Phase Dynamics

Fast-phase dynamics were studied using a tracer injected rapidly into the celiac artery through a femoral catheter. Radiograms of spleen, precordium, and liver were obtained in the same manner and then subjected to analysis[12]. In the fast-phase analysis, the dynamics of X-1 and X-2 were used but those of X-3 were excluded for technical reasons (Fig. 3, left).

In the analytic procedure, the transfer function of the heart-lung system to the spleen $H(t)$ was computed using a pair of radiograms—— precordium $X_1(t)$ as input and spleen $Y_1(t)$ as output taken after intravenous injection (Fig. 4, upper). These data were used to precisely evaluate the recirculation component $Y_2(t)$ in the radiosplenogram taken after intra-arterial injection. The following equations were used:

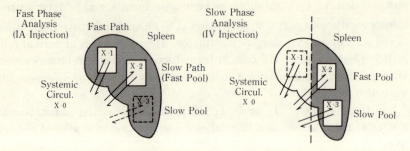

Fig. 3. Measurement and analysis of fast and slow dynamics.

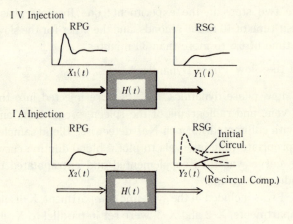

Fig. 4. Identification of recirculation component.

$$Y_1(t) = \int_0^t H(\tau) X_1(t-\tau) d\tau,$$

$$Y_2(t) = \int_0^t H(\tau) X_2(t-\tau) d\tau,$$

where $X_2(t)$ was the radiogram of the precordium after intra-arterial injection. The initial circulation component was then identified by subtracting the recirculation component from the original radiosplenogram. An analog simulation technique, the circuit of which is shown in Figure 5, was applied to compute the results (Fig. 7).

Because the dynamics of X-2 are included in both the fast and slow

Application of Compartmental Model of Spleen Hemodynamics

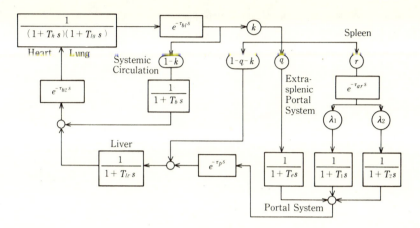

Fig. 5. Block diagram for analog computation.

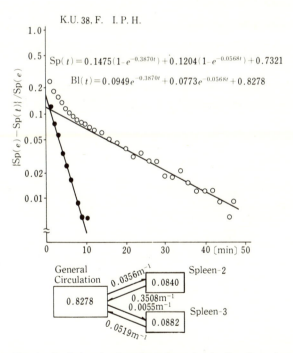

Fig. 6. Analysis of spleen hemodynamics in the slow phase (^{51}Cr-RBC).

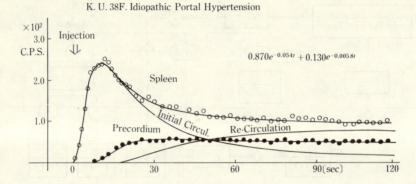

Fig. 7. Analysis of radiosplenogram by analog simulation ^{51}Cr-RBC into the splenic artery.

phases, the value computed by compartmental analysis (Fig. 6) was used as the output rate constant for X-2 (Fig. 7).

4.1.3 Overall Characterization

The overall characterization of splenic circulation was determined from the analysis of fast-and slow-phase dynamics (Fig. 8).

4.1.4 Other Parameters Related to Spleen Hemodynamics

Splenic blood flow was determined by measuring the washout rate of

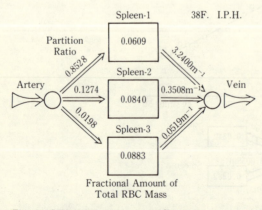

Fig. 8. Splenic hemodynamics of ^{51}Cr-RBC.

^{133}Xe from the spleen after its intra-arterial injection, and by measuring the maximum clearance rate of ^{51}Cr- or ^{99m}Tc-labeled heat-denatured red cells, λ_{-f}, in the circulation after intravenous injection[11,13].

The volume of the spleen was assessed quantitatively by scintigraphy and expressed as the splenic volume index in cm^3/kg of body weight[3,13].

Circulating blood volume, red cell mass, and the survival of labeled cells were measured with ^{51}Cr red cells. The destruction rate of the labeled cells, λ_{-d}, was determined as the initial rate of decline in ^{51}Cr red cells immediately after equilibrium, following their intravenous administration[13].

The mean life span (MLS) of red cells was calibrated according to the formula:

$$MLS = 1/(\lambda_{-d} - \lambda_{-e}),$$

where λ_{-e} is the rate at which ^{51}Cr was eluted from the red cells.

4.2 RESULTS AND COMMENTS

Results of 111 studies of spleen hemodynamics in 74 patients were classified into seven groups as shown in Table 1.

4.2.1 Implication of Fast-Flow Compartment

From the data presented in Table 1, the characteristics of the fast compartment can be summarized as follows:

1. Among different disease groups, there was no significant difference in the average value of the partition ratio for autologous red cells, β_1, into the first compartment.

2. There was a close relationship between the exit rate constants of this compartment for red cells, β_{10}, and for plasma, α_{10}, in an individual group and total groups alike.

These data indicate that approximately 80% of red cells from the splenic artery enter the fast compartment, irrespective of the disease, and leave there with plasma without much impediment. For example, HS cells are considered to pass through a particularly rough sieve in their own spleen, since β_1 for normal cells (N-C) was significantly greater than that for autogeneous HS cells (A-C), while β_1 for HS cells in normal spleen (Cont. SP HS-C) was remarkably smaller than β_1 for HS cells in autologous HS spleen.

Considering the findings of perfusion experiments in the dog spleen, it is reasonable to assume that splenic blood flow is regulated to maintain a certain level through this first compartment as a fast path.

Table 1. Analyses of spleen hemodynamics

	n	λ_{-t}	β_1	β_2	β_3	β_{10}	β_{20}	β_{30}	V_0	V_1	V_2	V_3
Control	(10)	0.0397 ±0.0066	0.789 0.097	0.211 ±0.097	nil	6.654 ±3.108	1.176 ±0.368	—	—	—	—	—
HS A-C	(15)	0.1637 ±0.0487	0.775 ±0.071	0.205 ±0.068	0.020 ±0.009	5.414 ±1.977	0.438 ±0.132	0.053 ±0.024	0.875 ±0.050	0.022 ±0.010	0.069 ±0.027	0.056 ±0.026
N-C	(14)	0.1690 ±0.0476	0.815 ±0.060	0.177 ±0.058	0.006 ±0.008	5.775 ±3.232	0.614 ±0.242	0.087 ±0.023	0.933 ±0.032	0.026 ±0.012	0.051 ±0.024	0.016 ±0.013
Cont. Sp HS-C	(1)	0.0422	0.481	0.260	0.259	4.080	0.436	0.054	0.815	0.004	0.021	0.165
AIHA	(16)	0.1458 ±0.0620	0.804 ±0.040	0.186 ±0.087	0.010 ±0.008	4.286 ±1.605	0.755 ±0.459	0.066 ±0.042	0.933 ±0.043	0.028 ±0.017	0.041 ±0.022	0.026 ±0.023
CS	(39)	0.2392 ±0.0761	0.791 ±0.085	0.197 ±0.083	0.012 ±0.008	2.277 ±0.803	0.608 ±0.161	0.063 ±0.019	0.888 ±0.059	0.073 ±0.029	0.070 ±0.035	0.042 ±0.031
Diff. Shunt	(16)	0.0127 ±0.0506	0.0111 ±0.1023	−0.0111 ±0.1010	−0.0001 ±0.0052	0.3328 ±0.5954	−0.0435 ±0.1700	−0.0033 ±0.0302	−0.0055 ±0.0475	−0.0064 ±0.0243	0.0010 ±0.0269	0.0047 ±0.0250

	SVI	Volume Ratio	B.V.	λ_{-d}	K_{-xe}	$1/\tau_p$	α_{10}	
Control	4.5 ± 0.8	—	68.7 ± 5.9	0.0243 ±0.0017	1.364 ±0.240	4.064 ±0.660	5.514 ±1.123	A-C, N-C: autogeneous HS cells and normal cells in the HS spleen.
HS A-C	24.0 ± 8.8	—	68.7 ± 9.2	0.0977 ±0.0346	1.065 ±0.269	4.929 ±0.601	6.931 ±2.457	AIHA: acquired autoimmune hemolytic anemia.
N-C	24.7 ± 8.7	—	62.6 ± 5.2	0.0288 ±0.0046	1.082 ±0.272	4.969 ±0.604	7.044 ±2.576	CS: congestive splenomegalies associated with portal hypertension.
Cont. Sp HS-C	5.6	—	82.6	0.2567	1.165	4.591	6.240	Diff. Shunt: difference induced by portal-systemic shunt operation.
AIHA	15.4 ± 4.3	—	64.4 ± 8.6	0.1404 ±0.1370	1.347 ±0.270	4.186 ±0.549	5.970 ±1.896	n: number of cases
CS	29.0 ± 8.5	—	84.6 ±12.7	0.0383 ±0.0092	1.042 ±0.289	2.634 ±1.041	3.691 ±1.894	
Diff. Shunt	− 4.31 ± 8.36	− 7.6 ±35.8	− 0.63 ± 8.60	0.0079 ±0.0075	0.1870 ±0.2888	0.6224 ±1.0520	0.999 ±2.063	

4.2.2. Slow Dynamics Compartment and Red Cell Destruction

To clarify the role of splenic hemodynamics in red cell destruction, regression analysis in which the destruction rate of red cells (λ_{-d}) was an objective variable and splenic hemodynamic parameters were explanatory variables, was carried out by selecting variables by the stepwise procedure[14]. Table 2 shows a standardized regression coefficient for each selected variable and the multiple correlation coefficient between predicted and observed values.

The highest correlation coefficient obtained was in the HS group in which changes in splenic hemodynamics comprised 90% of the accelerating factor of red cell destruction. The cellular factor attributable to an inherited defect in the HS cell was elucidated by calculating the regression value of the difference in red cell destruction (A-N Dif.) between HS and normal cells in the same HS spleen on the difference of hemodynamic parameters between the two kinds of cells.

In some cases of congestive splenomegaly associated with portal hypertension, a porta-systemic shunting operation induced excessive hemolysis even though the splenomegaly was partially improved. These cases provided examples for analyzing splenic factor. The regression

Table 2. Analysis of RBC destruction

	n	Mult. Corr.	Blood Volume	Spleen Size	Spl. Flow	Plasma
HS	15	0.956	—	—	—	$0.235(1/\tau_p)$
A-N Dif.	14	0.880	—	0.583(SVI)	$-0.439(\lambda_{-f})$	—
AIHA	16	0.613	-0.364(BV)	—	—	—
CS	39	0.787	—	—	$0.300(\lambda_{-f})$	$-0.319(1/\tau_p)$
IPH	20	0.752	—	—	$0.367(K_{-xe})$	—
LC	19	0.934	0.438(BV)	—	—	—
Diff. Shunt	16	0.893	—	—	—	$1.208(1/\tau_p)$

			RBC Dynamics		
	n	Part. Ratio	Inflow	Outflow	Comp. Size
HS	15	—	—	$-0.355(\beta_{20})$	$-0.892(V_0)$
A-N Dif.	14	—	—	$-0.265(\beta_{30})$	$0.684(V_3)$
AIHA	16	$0.523(\beta_3)$	—	—	$-0.279(V_2)$
CS	39	—	—	—	$-0.462(V_0)$
IPH	20	—	—	$0.454(\beta_{30})$	$0.586(V_2)$
LC	19	—	—	—	$0.239(V_1)$ $0.300(V_2)$
Diff. Shunt	16	$0.527(\beta_2)$	$-0.2921(\beta_{03})$	$-0.471(\beta_{20})$	—

analysis was again made to evaluate the influence of postoperative changes in spleen hemodynamics on the red cell destruction rate (Diff. Shunt in Table 2).

Accelerating factors for red cell destruction commonly found in these and other disease groups were: (a) the increase in the partition ratio of red cells to the slow pool, β_3, with reduced exit rate, β_{30}, and (b) the increase in the volume of this pool, V_3, irrespective of plasma flow, α_{10}, or $1/\tau_p$, i.e., the reciprocal of plasma mean transit time.

4.2.3 Morphologic Counterpart of the Dynamic Compartment

To complete our work, it was considered necessary and important to look for anatomic counterparts of the compartments defined from the hemodynamic standpoint.

For these studies, spleens sufficiently perfused immediately after they were removed from patients with idiopathic thrombocytopenic purpura were used. Autologous red cells were denatured so that at least 50% of them would be diverted from the fast passage because they were predisposed to splenic trapping[5,13]. The cells were infused gently into the spleen, which was fixed, and silver stained specimens were examined histologically.

The newly infused cells were not distributed uniformly in the red pulp. Some were lined up as if they were routed preferentially from the arterial ending to a certain selected locus of the sinus wall, where several cells were passing through the wall into the sinus space. The loci were not necessarily adjacent to the arterial endings, nor were the routes necessarily the shortest. It is reasonable to assume that these routes are the preferential ones[15], corresponding to the dynamics of the first compartment.

Other cells were seen to deviate from these routes and to scatter in the mesh work of the pulp cords as though searching for another exit. Their dynamics should be allotted to the second intermediate compartment[15].

Spleens which were removed from patients with hemolytic anemia and in which spleen hemodynamics had been measured in vivo preoperatively, were examined by histometry. Red cells surrounding a single sinus wall were counted, and the count was corrected with reference to the rectangular section to the wall. Corrected counts from about 70 sinuses were averaged. This average number of surrounding cells correlated significantly with the dynamics parameters of the third compartment, the exit rate constant for the cells, β_{30}[15], and the fractional amount of cells in this compartment, V_3. Therefore, cells situated on or around the sinus walls were considered to reflect the dynamics of the third, slow pool, compartment.

4.2.4 Functional Interpretation

Results of kinetic analyses indicated that red cells in the intermediate and, especially, in the slow compartments were in a highly concentrated state due to plasma depletion. In this 'bottle neck' state, blood viscosity becomes infinite. From the metabolic aspect, the assumed state of low metabolic substate, low pO_2 and low pH cause the cells to become more rigid as they loose their membrane flexibility and intracellular fluidity. This condition would make it more difficult for the cells to pass through the narrow slits in the sinus wall, which requires extreme cell-deformation.

This concept was supported by studies on red cells collected in the early and late phases of perfusion from spleens removed from patients with hemolytic anemia or thrombocytopenia. The 'late phase' cells caused a decrease in the resistance to hypotonicity, thus reflecting a loss of membrane flexibility. By scanning electron microscopy, these cells contained a large number of abnormal cells, such as stomatocytes and echinocytes, and fragmented cells.

Repeated and prolonged exposure to this unfavorable environment, as described above, will reduce cell viability and finally lead to cellular destruction in the spleen or elsewhere in the circulation.

5. CONCLUSION

Spleen hemodynamics, examined by perfusion experiments, were well represented by the sum of exponential components corresponding to the fast and slow dynamic phases. The red cell dynamics were represented by a first order system with three compartments, fast, intermediate and slow, and the plasma dynamics by a first order 2-compartment system.

Measurements and analyses in spleen hemodynamics were carried out *in vivo* with plasma and red cell tracers by using different methods for the fast and slow dynamic phases. Utilizing our model, the results could be explained comprehensively with the overall characteristics of spleen hemodynamics.

The dynamics of the fast compartment, in which about 80% of the red cells in the arterial inflow participated irrespective of diseases, were supposed to be regulated so as to maintain flow rate. In the intermediate and slow compartments, red cells were delayed in flow rate with a reduced ratio of plasma, and subjected to metabolic stress.

Multiple regression analysis on the dynamics parameters revealed a close relationship between red cell kinetics in the slow compartment and their destruction rate.

Several experiments were done to define the anatomic counterparts of these compartments and to obtain both morphologic and functional confirmation of the concepts derived from kinetic studies.

This dynamics study revealed that the fast and slow phases cover the time order from several seconds to an hour, as demonstrated by experimental studies using the isolated spleen[10]. Our *in vivo* method not only elucidates the dynamics under physiologic conditions, but also permits repeated study to follow changes in a disease state, or to evaluate the effect of treatment.

REFERENCES

1. Weiss, L.: The spleen. In *The Blood Cell and Hemopoietic Tissues,* 545-573, McGraw Hill Inc. New York, 1977.
2. Harris, I.M., McAlister, J.and Prankerd, T.A.J.: Splenomegaly and circulating red cells. *Brit.J. Haematol.* 4: 97-102, 1958.
3. Takahashi, Y.: Clinical studies on sequestration function of the spleen, I.Circulatory dynamics of the spleen with special reference to its role in red cell destruction. II. Quantitative estimation of the spleen volume by scintigraphy and examination of its function with damaged cell clearance. *Acta Haematol. Jap.* 30: 83-145, 1967.
4. Jandle, J.H. & Aster, R.H.: Increased splenic pooling and the pathogenesis of hypersplenism. *Am.J. Med. Sci.* 253: 383-398, 1967.
5. Takahashi, Y., Kariyone, S., Uyama, C. et al.: Studies on splenic hemodynamics and blood cell destruction by simulation analysis of radiosplenogram. *Proceedings of the first world congress of nuclear medicine,* 97-101. World federation of nuclear medicine and biology, Tokyo, 1974.
6. Chen, L.T. & Weiss, L: The roll of the sinus wall in the passage of erythrocytes through the spleen. *Blood* 41: 529-537, 1973.
7. Rappaport, H.: The pathologic anatomy of the spleen red pulp. In *Milz/Spleen,* edited by K. Lennert and D. Harms. Springer-Verlag, Berlin, 24-41, 1970.
8. Schmid-Schoenbein, H.: Hemorheological aspects of splenic function. In *Milz/Spleen* (ibid.), 67-80.
9. Bowdler, A.J.: Theoretical considerations of measurement of the splenic red cell pool. *Clin. Sci.* 23: 181-196, 1962.
10. Levesque, M.J. & Groom, A.C.: Washout kinetics of red cells and plasma in the spleen. *Am. J.Physiol.* 231: 1665-1671, 1976.
11. Kariyone, S. & Takahashi, Y.: Circulatory dynamics and function of the spleen. *J.Clin. Sci.* 8: 379-389, 1972 (in Japanese).
12. Takahashi, Y., Uyama, C. & Sohma, T.: Analysis of splenic circulation model using radiosplenogram. I. Simulation experiment. *Jap. J. MEBE* 11: 163-172, 1973 (in Japanese).
13. Takahashi, Y.: Determination of red cell survival and examination of the splenic and other

reticuloendothelial functions. *Jpn. J. Clin. Path.* 21 : 329-340, 1973 (in Japanese).
14 Draper, N.R. & Smith, H : Selecting the "best" regression equation. In *Applied Regression Analysis*. John Wiley & Sons, Inc. New York, Ch. 6, 163-215, 1966.
15 Takahashi, Y : Analysis of the spleen hemodynamics and red cell destruction, Symposium on hemolysis and spleen. *Jpn. J. Clin. Haematol.* 22 : 592-607, 1981 (in Japanese).

14
MULTI-COMPARTMENTAL SYSTEM WITH STOCHASTIC INPUT——MATHEMATICAL FORMULATION BY THE ITO CALCULUS AND ITS APPLICATION TO HEALTH PHYSICS

Shinobu Tatsunami, Nagasumi Yago and Nobuo Fukuda

1. INTRODUCTION

Tissue concentrations of fallouts as well as of naturally occurring radionuclides usually vary widely among individuals. From the standpoint of the systems theory, two major factors may be responsible for this variation: (a) the fluctuation of transfer coefficients and (b) the daily intake of radionuclide, i.e., the stochastic input.

As exemplified by their Monte-Carlo simulation, Matthies et al.[1] successfully demonstrated that the variation in ^{137}Cs concentrations in the pasture-cow-milk food chain depends on the fluctuation of its transfer coefficients.

However, we believe that cases exist wherein the stochasticity of inputs becomes the major cause for the variation in tissue concentrations of radionuclide, while transfer coefficients remain rather constant for long periods. Such cases would most probably be realized especially when very small amounts of radionuclides are taken up daily under normal dietary conditions.

We have thus explored, using Ito calculus, the possibility that the fluctuation in tissue radionuclide concentrations is the result of continuous but stochastic inputs. We describe the derivation of rate equations with stochastic inputs from the system exterior and the results of its application to ^{210}Po metabolism in the human body.

2. THEORETICAL

2.1 DEFINITION OF THE MULTI-COMPARTMENTAL SYSTEM STUDIED

A multi-compartmental system composed of n compartments is discussed. Each compartment is connected to all others and receives stochastically fluctuating inputs from outside this particular system (Fig. 1).

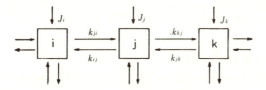

Fig. 1. The multi-compartmental system with stochastic input J from outside the system. Each compartment is connected linearly with the others through the transfer coefficient denoted by k.

2.2 MATHEMATICAL FORMULATION OF THE STOCHASTIC INPUTS FROM OUTSIDE THE MULTI-COMPARTMENTAL SYSTEM

In the multi-compartmental system, stochastically fluctuating inputs, $J_i(t)$, into the ith compartment from outside this particular system at time t are assumed to be composed of two terms: its own expected value, $\text{Exp}[J_i(t)]$, and the deviation, $F_i(t)$, which changes stochastically around the expected value. Thus, $J_i(t)$ can be expressed by Eq. 1

$$J_i(t) = \text{Exp}[J_i(t)] + F_i(t). \qquad (1)$$

Further, the term $\text{Exp}[J_i(t)]$ is assumed to be approximated by a continuous function, $f_i(t)$, as follows:

$$\text{Exp}[J_i(t)] = f_i(t). \qquad (2)$$

With respect to $F_i(t)$, the mathematical condition under which $\text{Exp}[F_i(t)]$ should be zero, according to Eq. 1, is noted. One way to satisfy this condition would be to assume that $F_i(t)$ is the product of a continuous function, $\sigma_i(t)$, and the white noise, $h(t, w)$, as expressed in Eq. 3,

$$F_i(t) = h(t, w)\sigma_i(t), \tag{3}$$

where w is the symbol for stochasticity.

By definition,

$$\mathrm{Exp}[h(t, w)] = 0 \tag{4}$$

satisfies the above-mentioned mathematical equation.

Substituting Eqs. 2 and 3 in Eq. 1 gives Eq. 5 for the mathematical formulation of stochastic inputs into the ith compartment from the system exterior:

$$J_i(t) = f_i(t) + h(t, w)\sigma_i(t). \tag{5}$$

2.3 RATE EQUATIONS CONTAINING STOCHASTIC INPUTS AND THEIR SOLUTIONS

The differential equation that describes the rate at which the amount of the compartment of the ith compartment changes at time t, denoted by $x_i(t)$, may be written as follows:

$$\frac{dx_i(t)}{dt} = (f_i(t) + h(t, w)\sigma_i(t)) + \sum_{j \neq i} k_{ij} x_j(t) - (\sum_{j \neq i} k_{ji}) \cdot x_i(t) - k_{0i} x_i(t),$$

where k_{ij} denotes the transfer coefficient from the jth to the ith compartment, and k_{0i}, the collective rate constant for the decrease in $x_i(t)$ through its own decay within the ith compartment and its excretion to the outside of the system.

Thus, we have the following set of simultaneous differential

$$\frac{d}{dt}\begin{bmatrix} x_1(t) \\ x_2(t) \\ \vdots \\ x_n(t) \end{bmatrix} = \begin{bmatrix} f_1(t) \\ f_2(t) \\ \vdots \\ f_n(t) \end{bmatrix} + h(t, w)\begin{bmatrix} \sigma_1(t) \\ \sigma_2(t) \\ \vdots \\ \sigma_n(t) \end{bmatrix} - K\begin{bmatrix} x_1(t) \\ x_2(t) \\ \vdots \\ x_n(t) \end{bmatrix} \tag{6}$$

equations for all compartments, from the first to the nth, of the system in which K is the n-n matrix composed of transfer coefficients between the compartments. Therefore, components of the matrix are defined as follows:

$$K_{ij} = -k_{ij}$$
$$K_{ii} = \sum_{j \neq i} k_{ji} + k_{0i}.$$

Using Ito's method[2,3], Eq. 6 may be transformed into the following

$$d\begin{bmatrix} x_1(t) \\ x_2(t) \\ \vdots \\ x_n(t) \end{bmatrix} = \left(\begin{bmatrix} f_1(t) \\ f_2(t) \\ \vdots \\ f_n(t) \end{bmatrix} - K \begin{bmatrix} x_1(t) \\ x_2(t) \\ \vdots \\ x_n(t) \end{bmatrix} \right) dt + \begin{bmatrix} \sigma_1(t) \\ \sigma_2(t) \\ \vdots \\ \sigma_n(t) \end{bmatrix} dB_t, \qquad (7)$$

where B_t is the time integral of the white noise, or what is conventionally referred to as the Brownian motion,

$$B_t = \int_0^t h(t', w) dt'.$$

Multiplying e^{Kt}, we obtain Eq. 8,

$$d\left(e^{Kt} \begin{bmatrix} x_1(t) \\ x_2(t) \\ \vdots \\ x_n(t) \end{bmatrix} \right) = e^{Kt} \begin{bmatrix} f_1(t) \\ f_2(t) \\ \vdots \\ f_n(t) \end{bmatrix} dt + e^{Kt} \begin{bmatrix} \sigma_1(t) \\ \sigma_2(t) \\ \vdots \\ \sigma_n(t) \end{bmatrix} dB_t. \qquad (8)$$

Integrating Eq. 8 under the initial condition of $x_i(t) = 0$ $(i = 1, \cdots, n)$, yields Eq. 9,

$$\begin{bmatrix} x_1(t) \\ x_2(t) \\ \vdots \\ x_n(t) \end{bmatrix} = \int_0^t e^{-K(t-t')} \begin{bmatrix} f_1(t') \\ f_2(t') \\ \vdots \\ f_n(t') \end{bmatrix} dt'$$

$$+ \int_0^t e^{-K(t-t')} \begin{bmatrix} \sigma_1(t') \\ \sigma_2(t') \\ \vdots \\ \sigma_n(t') \end{bmatrix} h(t', w) dt'. \qquad (9)$$

2.4 ALGORITHM

For practical purposes, Eq. 9 may be rewritten as follows:

The deterministic component of the input, that is the vector $\vec{f_i}(t')$, may be written, as in Eq. 10, using the unit vector $\vec{i_i}$,

$$\begin{bmatrix} f_1(t') \\ f_2(t') \\ \vdots \\ f_n(t') \end{bmatrix} = \sum_i f_i(t') \vec{i_i}. \qquad (10)$$

The unit vector $\vec{i_i}$ in Eq. 10 is defined in such a way that the ith component is unity, while all others are zero. The unit vector may be expanded by the eigen vector of K with $_ic_j$ as the expansion coefficient,

$$\vec{i_i} = \sum_j {}_ic_j \vec{a_j}$$

where $\vec{a_j}$ is the jth eigen vector of K

$$K\vec{a_j} = \lambda_j \vec{a_j} . \tag{11}$$

Thus, Eq. 10 may be rewritten as

$$\begin{bmatrix} f_1(t') \\ f_2(t') \\ \vdots \\ f_n(t') \end{bmatrix} = \sum_m f_m(t')(\sum_m {}_m c_k \vec{a_k}) . \tag{12}$$

Using Eqs. 11 and 12, we obtain Eq. 13 for the first deterministic term of Eq. 9:

$$\int_0^t e^{-K(t-t')} \begin{bmatrix} f_1(t') \\ f_2(t') \\ \vdots \\ f_n(t') \end{bmatrix} dt' = \int_0^t \sum_m f_m(t')(\sum_k e^{-\lambda_k(t-t')} {}_m c_k \vec{a_k}) dt' . \tag{13}$$

Through procedures similar to those described above, the second term of Eq. 9 on stochasticity may be rewritten as follows:

$$\int_0^t e^{-K(t-t')} \begin{bmatrix} \sigma_1(t') \\ \sigma_2(t') \\ \vdots \\ \sigma_n(t') \end{bmatrix} h(t', w) dt'$$

$$= \int_0^t h(t', w)(\sum_m \sigma_m(t')(\sum_k e^{-\lambda_k(t-t')} {}_m \dot{c}_k \vec{a_k})) dt' . \tag{14}$$

Substituting Eqs. 13 and 14 into Eq. 9, yields Eq. 15 for the ith compartment,

$$x_i(t) = \int_0^t (\sum_m f_m(t')(\sum_k e^{-\lambda_k(t-t')} {}_m c_k a_{ik})) dt'$$
$$+ \int_0^t h(t', w)(\sum_m \sigma_m(t')(\sum_k e^{-\lambda_k(t-t')} {}_m \dot{c}_k a_{ik})) dt' , \tag{15}$$

where a_{ik} is the ith component of the vector $\vec{a_k}$.

The expected value of $x_i(t)$ may be obtained as follows by using the definition of the white noise in Eq. 4,

$$\mathrm{Exp}[x_i(t)] = \int_0^t \sum_m f_m(t')(\sum_k e^{-\lambda_k(t-t')}{}_mC_k a_{ik})dt'. \tag{16}$$

The variance-covariance matrix element denoted as V_{ij} is given by Eq. 17:

$$\begin{aligned}V_{ij}(t) &\equiv \mathrm{Exp}[(x_i(t) - \mathrm{Exp}[x_i(t)])(x_j(t) - \mathrm{Exp}[x_j(t)])] \\ &= \mathrm{Exp}\Big[\int_0^t (h(t', w) \cdot \sum_m \sigma_m(t')(\sum_k e^{-\lambda_k(t-t')}{}_mC_k a_{ik}))dt' \\ &\quad \cdot \int_0^t (h(t'', w) \cdot \sum_m \sigma_m(t'')(\sum_k e^{-\lambda_k(t-t'')}{}_mC_k a_{jk}))dt''\Big]. \end{aligned} \tag{17}$$

The auto-correlation function of the white noise is known to be related to Dirac's delta function with the power of the white noise $\gamma/2$,

$$\mathrm{Exp}[h(t,w)h(t',w)] = \frac{1}{2}\gamma\delta(t-t').$$

We normalize $\gamma/2$ to unity temporarily, or incorporate the contribution of the power of the white noise into the function $\sigma_i(t)$ so that Eq. 17 is finally written as:

$$\begin{aligned}V_{ij}(t) = \int_0^t &((\sum_m \sigma_m(t')(\sum_k e^{-\lambda_k(t-t')}{}_mC_k a_{ik})) \\ &\cdot (\sum_m \sigma_m(t')(\sum_k e^{-\lambda_k(t-t')}{}_mC_k a_{jk})))dt'.\end{aligned} \tag{18}$$

2.5 SYSTEM WITH STATIONARY STOCHASTIC INPUTS FROM SYSTEM EXTERIOR

Based on Eqs. 16 and 18, a simple yet often-encountered system is considered, i.e., one with stationary stochastic input from an external source. In this case, $\vec{f_i}$ and $\vec{\sigma_i}$ may be expanded with the eigen vectors of K:

$$\begin{bmatrix} f_1 \\ f_2 \\ \vdots \\ f_n \end{bmatrix} = \sum_k d_k \vec{a_k} \quad (19), \qquad \begin{bmatrix} \sigma_1 \\ \sigma_2 \\ \vdots \\ \sigma_n \end{bmatrix} = \sum_k g_k \vec{a_k}, \tag{20}$$

where d_k and g_k are expressed respectively, as follows:

$$d_k = \sum_m f_m \, {}_m C_k, \tag{21}$$

$$g_k = \sum_m \sigma_m \, {}_m C_k. \tag{22}$$

Substituting Eqs. 19 through 22 into Eqs. 16 and 18, yields:

$$\mathrm{Exp}[x_i(t)] = \sum_k \frac{1-e^{-\lambda_k t}}{\lambda_k} d_k a_{ik}, \tag{23}$$

$$V_{ij}(t) = \sum_k \sum_m \frac{1-e^{-(\lambda_k+\lambda_m)t}}{\lambda_k+\lambda_m} g_k a_{ik} g_m a_{jm}. \tag{24}$$

3. ESTIMATION OF AMOUNTS OF ^{210}Po ACCUMULATED IN THE HUMAN BODY

One of the most common cases in which stochastic inputs are encountered is the intake of foods containing the widely distributed radionuclide ^{210}Po.[4] This particular radionuclide is mainly derived from the decay of ^{238}U and partly from airborne fallout. It accumulates in human tissues due to its affinity for cellular proteins and its relatively long half life of 138.4 days.

Human ^{210}Po metabolism has been modeled by Bernard[5] as a 2-compartment system with the transfer coefficients shown in Figure 2.

Thus, the matrix of transfer coefficients is written as follows:

$$K = \begin{bmatrix} 0.025+0.685+\lambda_p & -0.703 \\ -0.685 & 0.703+\lambda_p \end{bmatrix}, \tag{25}$$

where λ_p is the physical decay constant of ^{210}Po.

Then, the average value for ^{210}Po in the reference man[6] is assumed to be the continuous function of input defined in Eq. 2, i.e., $f_1(t) = 3.2$ pCi/day. Secondly, assuming that the probability distribution of ^{210}Po intake is described by the standard Gaussian distribution, the stochastic input can be written as follows:

$$\begin{bmatrix} J_1 \\ J_2 \end{bmatrix} = \begin{bmatrix} 3.2 \\ 0 \end{bmatrix} + h(t,w) \begin{bmatrix} \sqrt{3.2} \\ 0 \end{bmatrix}. \tag{26}$$

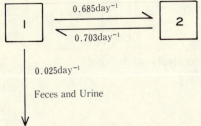

Fig. 2. 2-compartment model for ^{210}Po metabolism in humans.

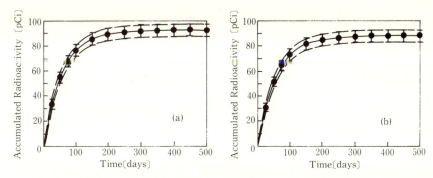

Fig. 3. Radioactivities of ^{210}Po (pCi) accumulated in compartments 1 (shown in (a)) and 2 (shown in (b)) of the reference man of Figure 2. Solid lines represent values of $\text{Exp}[x_i(t)]$ ($i=1, 2$) calculated by Eq. 23 and broken lines those of the standard deviation of the values of $\text{Exp}[x_i(t)]$ by Eq. 24. Solid circles show the values of $\text{Exp}[x_i(t)]$ and bars the standard deviation computed by the Monte-Carlo simulation described in Section 4.

Substituting Eqs. 25 and 26 into Eqs. 23 and 24, both the expected value and variance of the amount of ^{210}Po at any time point in each of the two compartments can be calculated.

4. VALIDITY TEST OF VARIANCE CALCULATION THROUGH MONTE-CARLO SIMULATION

Whether the calculation of expected value and variance by the present method properly represents the real system was tested by a computer experiment using the ^{210}Po intake by humans. By the inverse Gaussian distribution method compiled into a FORTRAN program (Code RANDON of the Univac, Japan), 500 random numbers with both mean and variance of 3.2, were first generated in the UNIVAC computer (1100/model 21).

Because each of these random numbers was used as the daily input of ^{210}Po from the system exterior into compartment 1 of Figure 2, the following equation (27) was used to compute the amounts of ^{210}Po in each of the two compartments under the condition that both of them were initially empty.

$$\begin{bmatrix} x_1(t) \\ x_2(t) \end{bmatrix} = \int_0^t e^{-K(t-t')} \begin{bmatrix} J_1(t') \\ 0 \end{bmatrix} dt' . \qquad (27)$$

In practice, Eq. 27 was approximated in the computer by Eq. 28, and the amounts of ^{210}Po, in terms of pCi, were computed from 1 through 500 days ($n=1\sim500$) by substituting the random numbers into the term $J_1(t_k)\Delta t$,

$$\begin{bmatrix}x_1(t_n)\\x_2(t_n)\end{bmatrix} \simeq \begin{bmatrix} \sum_{m=1}^{2}\left(\frac{d_m a_{1m}}{\lambda_m}(1-e^{-\lambda_m \Delta t})\left(\sum_{k=1}^{n}J_1(t_k)\Delta t e^{-\lambda_m(t_n-t_k)}\right)\right) \\ \sum_{m=1}^{2}\left(\frac{d_m a_{2m}}{\lambda_m}(1-e^{-\lambda_m \Delta t})\left(\sum_{k=1}^{n}J_1(t_k)\Delta t e^{-\lambda_m(t_n-t_k)}\right)\right) \end{bmatrix} \quad (28)$$

After the computation was repeated 500 times, the ensemble average and variance were calculated. The results were practically the same as those obtained in the preceeding section (all values were consistent within the relative difference of 0.5%). The values calculated using Eq. 28 are shown in Figure 3 as solid circles (ensemble average) and bars ($\pm$ standard deviation) every 50 days.

5. DISCUSSION

One of the most unique features of the present study was the derivation of a mathematical formula for the stochastic input into a system from the outside while transfer coefficients remained constant. The Ito calculus has thus been proved suitable for describing such a system and the analytical equations that resulted were easy to apply to practical situations, as illustrated by human ^{210}Po metabolism. As a matter of fact, the results computed by the present method were consistent with those generated by the computer experiment.

To further extend the present method, cases in which transfer coefficients fluctuate stochastically are currently being investigated.

ACKNOWLEDGMENT

We wish to express our sincere gratitude to Professor Masanao Hosoe, Institute for Atomic Energy, St. Paul's University, Yokosuka, Japan, for his valuable discussions, and to Mr. Akifusa Fujiki, St. Paul's University Computer Center, Tokyo, for his help in the present computations.

REFERENCES

1. Matthies, M., Eisfeld, K., Paretzke, H. et al.: Stochastic calculations for radiation risk assessment: A Monte-Carlo approach to the simulation of radiocesium transport in the pasture-cow-milk food chain. *Health Physics* 40: 764-769, 1981.
2. Ito, K.: Stochastic integral. *Proc. Imp. Acad. Japan* 20: 519-524, 1944.
3. Ito, K.: On stochastic differential equation. *Mem. Am. Math. Soc.* 4: 1-51, 1951.
4. Hill, C.R.: Polonium-210 in man. *Nature* 208: 423-428, 1965.
5. Bernard, S.R.: A metabolic model for polonium. *Health Physics* 36: 731-732, 1979.
6. International Commission on Radiological Protection: Report of the task group on reference man. ICRP Publication No. 23, Pergamon Press, Oxford and New York, 1975. p. 402.

15
OPTIMAL DRUG ADMINISTRATION BASED ON A COMPARTMENTAL SYSTEM

Hideo Kusuoka, Hajime Maeda, Shinzo Kodama, Michitoshi Inoue, Hiroshi Abe and Fumihiko Kajiya

1. INTRODUCTION

In recent years, compartmental systems have been used effectively as mathematical models for the distribution of drugs[1]. When a drug is to be administered, it is desirable, for therapeutic reasons, to maintain optimum amounts of the drug at target sites and, at the same time, minimize the total dose to be administered so as to reduce the risk of side effects. Conventional methods of drug administration in clinical practice do not always meet these conditions; methods that do are defined as "optimal drug administration."[2,3] In this chapter a linear compartmental system serves as a pharmacokinetic model and the problems of optimal drug administration are considered. Conventional methods for administering drugs are also evaluated based on theoretical results.

2. SOLUTION OF THE OPTIMAL DRUG ADMINISTRATION PROBLEM

In this section a non-oscillatory compartmental system is used as the pharmacokinetic model, and the problem of optimal drug administration solved by applying a solution algorithm of optimization in a non-oscillatory compartmental system. The properties of optimal drug administration are also discussed, using a 2-compartment model.

2.1 DESCRIPTION OF THE MODEL FOR PHARMACOKINETICS

To evaluate the distribution of a drug in the human body, a linear time-invariant non-oscillatory compartmental system (Fig. 1) is employed; compartment 1 is the gastrointestinal tract and compartment 2 the blood space (plasma space). The oral administration of a drug is regarded as impulsive input into the gastrointestinal tract, i.e., compartment 1. When the amount $\delta_i (i=0,\cdots,N)$ of drug is administered orally at time $\tau_i(i=0, \cdots, N)$, the plasma concentration of drug at time $t \in [\tau_k, \tau_{k+1}]$ is expressed as follows:

$$x(t) = \sum_{i=0}^{k} \delta_i h(t-\tau_i), \qquad (1)$$

where $h(t)$ is the impulse response of compartment 2, i.e., the concentration of drug in plasma after a unit dose is ingested.

The compartmental system is said to be non-oscillatory if the impulse response of the system has a unique maximum and is strictly monotone decreasing after reaching a peak. This property of non-oscillation is usually observed in a compartmental system that describes the kinetics of substances in a human body, especially of a drug.

2.2 OPTIMIZATION OF DRUG ADMINISTRATION

In this section, optimization of drug administration is considered, and said to be achieved when plasma levels of the drug are maintained as a required mode with a minimal total dose of drug so as to reduce side effects.

For therapeutic reasons, three types of constraints are assumed relative to plasma concentrations of drug.

Type 1: Plasma concentrations should be greater than the minimal effective plasma concentration of the drug (m_1), i.e.,

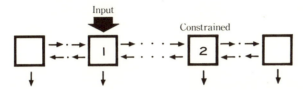

Fig. 1. A non-oscillatory linear compartmental system for pharmacokinetics in oral administration. Compartment 1 and Compartment 2 represent the gastrointestinal tract which receives inputs and the blood (plasma) space which is constrained, respectively.

$$x(t) \geq m_1, \quad t \in [\tau_1, \tau_N]. \tag{2}$$

Antibiotic is an example of this constraint.

Type 2 : Mean concentration should be maintained above a certain level (m_2), i.e.,

$$\text{mean}[x] = \frac{1}{\tau_i - \tau_{i-1}} \int_{\tau_{i-1}}^{\tau_i} x(t) dt \geq m_2, \quad \text{for} \quad i=1,\cdots,N. \tag{3}$$

For some drugs, plasma concentrations are a good indicator of their effects[4]. In this situation, to keep the drug's effect stable, the drug must be administered in such a way as to maintain a mean plasma concentration above a certain level.

Type 3 : The peak concentration between two consecutive administrations should exceed a certain level (m_3), i.e.,

$$\max_{\tau_i \leq t \leq \tau_{i+1}}[x] \geq m_3, \quad \text{for} \quad i=1,\cdots,N. \tag{4}$$

To minimize the total dosage of drug so as to reduce the possibility of side effects, the objective function to be minimized is defined as

$$g(u) = \sum_{i=0}^{N} \delta_i. \tag{5}$$

The optimal drug administration, therefore, involves finding a positive input sequence $u=(\delta_0, \delta_1,\cdots, \delta_N)^T$ which minimizes the objective function (5) under constraint (2), (3) or (4).

We have derived a theorem that gives an explicit formula of optimal input functions in a non-oscillatory compartmental system with a single input and a single constraint[5]. Optimal solutions are given by the following :

1. *Solution for type 1 constraint :*

$$u = m_1 M^{-1} e, \tag{6}$$

where $(M)_{ij} = h(\tau_i - \tau_{j-1}) \quad (i \geq j)$
$\phantom{(M)_{ij}} = 0 \quad (i < j),$

and $e = (1,\cdots, 1)^T$.

2. *Solution for type 2 constraint :*

$$u = m_2 M^{-1} e, \tag{7}$$

where

$$(M)_{ij} = \frac{1}{\tau_i - \tau_{i-1}} \int_{\tau_{i-1}}^{\tau_i} h(t - \tau_{j-1}) dt \quad (i \geq j)$$
$$= 0 \quad (i < j).$$

3. *Solution for type 3 constraint* :
The optimal solution is obtained by solving Eq. 8 successively.

$$\sum_{i=0}^{k} \delta_i h(t_k - \tau_i) = m_3, \quad \text{for} \quad k = 0, 1, \cdots, N, \tag{8}$$

where t_0 : the time that gives the maximum $h(t)$.
t_k : the time that gives the maximum $x(t)$ on $[\tau_k, \tau_{k+1}]$
$(k = 1, \cdots, N)$.

However, an approximate solution is given by

$$u = m_3 M^{-1} e, \tag{9}$$

where $(M)_{ij} = h(\tau_{i-1} - \tau_{j-1} + t_0) \quad (i \geq j)$
$= 0 \quad (i < j).$

2.3 PROPERTIES OF OPTIMAL DRUG ADMINISTRATION

In this section, a 2-compartment system is used as the model of pharmacokinetics and the properties of optimal drug administration, obtained theoretically in the previous section, are discussed.

To evaluate the distribution of drug in a human body, a system with two compartments is considered in this section (Fig. 2) ; the first compartment is the gastrointestinal tract and the second is an apparent distribution space containing blood space. The drug concentration in plasma after a single administration of a unit dose of drug—the impulse response $h(t)$ of the second compartment—is given by

$$h(t) = K(\exp(-\lambda_1 t) - \exp(-\lambda_2 t)), \tag{10}$$

where λ_1 and λ_2 $(0 < \lambda_1 < \lambda_2)$ are the eigenvalues of matrix A, and K is defined as $K = a_{21}/(\lambda_2 - \lambda_1)$. Matrix A is the compartment matrix of the system, i.e.,

$$A = \begin{bmatrix} -a_{21} & a_{12} \\ a_{21} & -(a_{12} + a_{02}) \end{bmatrix}. \tag{11}$$

Note that $h(t)$, given by Eq. 10, is non-oscillatory.

The property of optimal drug administration to maintain a minimal effective concentration in plasma, is discussed first. Suppose the drug is to

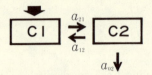

Fig. 2. A model for pharmacokinetics in oral administration to obtain the properties of optimal drug administration. C1 and C2 represent the gastrointestinal tract and an apparent space of drug distribution containing blood space, respectively. The rate constants a_{12}, a_{21}, and a_{02} are defined in the figure.

be administered at regular time intervals. If the time interval T is sufficiently large so that $\exp((\lambda_1-\lambda_2)T) \ll 1$, the optimal dose is nearly constant after the initial administration and $\delta_i (i=1,\cdots,N)$ is approximately given by

$$d = m_1(\exp(\lambda_1 T)-1)/K. \qquad (12)$$

That is, except for the initial dose (δ_0), the maintenance dose $(\delta_i, i=1,\cdots, N)$ is given by Eq. 12[5]. We examine the relationship between the total dosage (S_r) of drug to be used in a day for administration performed at regular intervals, and the total dosage (S_{ir}) required for irregular intervals. Within the range at which approximation Eq. 12 is satisfied, the total dosage in regular-interval administration, S_r, is calculated as

$$S_r = 24 m_1(\exp(\lambda_1 T)-1)/(KT) \qquad (13)$$

and we can show that

$$S_r < S_{ir} \qquad (14)$$

holds.

Next the relationship between the optimal dose and intervals to maintain mean concentrations of drug is examined. When the drug is given at regular intervals, the optimal maintenance dose can be shown to be nearly constant under mild conditions and is approximately given by

$$d = m_2 \lambda_1 \lambda_2 T/(K(\lambda_2-\lambda_1)). \qquad (15)$$

Moreover, we can show that the total dosage of drug to be used in a day is constant and independent of the mode of drug administration, i.e., independent of whether it is given at regular or irregular intervals and is given by

$$S = 24 m_2 \lambda_1 \lambda_2 / (K(\lambda_2 - \lambda_1)). \tag{16}$$

Finally, the relationship between optimal dose and interval required to maintain peak concentration of drug is examined. When the drug is given at regular intervals, the optimal maintenance dose is approximately given by

$$d = m_3 (\exp(\lambda_1 T) - 1)^\alpha / \{K(\xi^\alpha - \xi^\beta)(\exp(\lambda_2 T) - 1)^\beta\}, \tag{17}$$

where $\alpha = \lambda_1 / (\lambda_2 - \lambda_1)$, $\beta = \lambda_2 / (\lambda_2 - \lambda_1)$ and $\xi = \lambda_1 / \lambda_2$.
Therefore, the total dosage of drug to be used in a day is given by

$$S = 24 d / T. \tag{18}$$

3. ASSESSMENT OF CONVENTIONAL MODE OF DRUG ADMINISTRATION IN CLINICS

In Eqs. 12, 13, 15, 16, 17, and 18, we have given the properties of optimal drug dosage to maintain a plasma concentration of drug above a minimal effective level and to maintain the mean or peak concentration above a certain level. Figure 3 shows the relationship between optimal maintenance dose (d) and time interval (T) when the drug is given at regular time intervals. Figure 4 shows the relationship between optimal total dosage to be used in a day (S_r or S) and the time interval (T) for regular-interval administration.

Because the dose to be administered in the conventional manner is determined by dividing the total daily dosage equally, without considering the time intervals, these results suggest what follows.

When the minimal effective plasma concentration should be maintained, it can be done either by administering a variable dose at irregular time intervals or by administering a constant dose at regular intervals: when the drug is given at irregular intervals, the required dose should be varied, depending on the interval between drug administrations. These observations suggest that with the conventional mode of drug administration (e.g., three times a day after meals), each dose should be adjusted, depending on the length of the next interval. Consequently, in clinics the conventional mode agrees with optimal administration obtained theoretically only in the regular-interval case. This agreement does not hold for the irregular-interval administration. In administering a constant

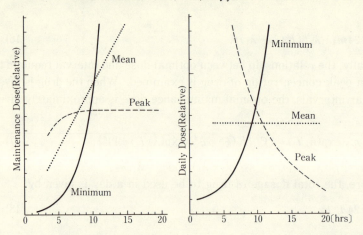

Fig. 3 (left) and *Fig. 4* (right). These figures show the relationship between the optimal maintenance dose and the length of the time intervals and the relationship between the optimal total dosage of drug to be used in a day and the length of the time intervals in regular-interval administration, respectively. The solid line represents the relationship when the plasma concentration of a drug is to be maintained above a minimal effective level. The dotted line and the broken line represent the dose required to maintain the mean and the peak concentration, respectively, above a certain level.

dose at regular intervals, it is suggested (Fig. 3) that the administration of drug at long time intervals is unfavorable, because each optimal dose increases exponentially with the length of the interval between doses. It is also unfavorable in view of the total dosage to be given in a day, as shown in Figure 4. From Eq. 14, it is found that the administration of drug at irregular intervals requires a total dosage greater than that prescribed when the drug is given at regular intervals. Therefore, the conventional mode is far from optimal drug administration, except when doses are given at regular intervals.

When the mean plasma concentration should be maintained, the variation of each optimal dose in the irregular interval administration is smaller than in the former case[6]. Moreover, the total dosage to be used in one day does not depend on the administration schedule; it is constant both in the regular and in the irregular interval administration. These results suggest that the conventional modes of drug administration in clinics is close to the optimal for maintaining the mean concentration.

When the peak concentration should be maintained, optimal maintenance doses are almost constant at longer time intervals. On the other hand, Figure 4 shows that the total daily dosage decreases with increasing time interval. Therefore, the conventional method correlates with optimal administration only when the peak drug concentration is maintained by administering doses at regular intervals.

Consequently, to maintain the mean plasma concentration the conventional mode of administration is nearly optimal. However, it is optimal to maintain neither the minimally effective concentration nor the peak concentration above a certain level. Thus, it is important to identify the constraint type to be observed when we schedule the dosage regimens of drug administration.

4. CONCLUSION

In this chapter, we have considered a non-oscillatory compartmental system for pharmacokinetics in oral administration. By applying the theorem which is concerned to impulsive optimal control of a non-oscillatory linear compartmental system, we have obtained the explicit formula of the optimal administration schedule. We next derived the specific characteristics of the optimal drug administration by using a two-compartment model for pharmacokinetics.

We have also evaluated the conventional mode of drug administration in clinics in view of the results theoretically obtained, and have shown that the conventional mode is close to the optimal administration in case of maintenance of mean plasma concentration, but far from the optimal administration except in the case of regular-interval administration when the purpose is to maintain either the minimal effective concentration or the peak concentration.

Thus, it is important to identify the constraint type to be observed when we schedule the dosage regimens of drug administration.

ACKNOWLEDGMENT

We are grateful to the IFIP, Elsevier North Holland Inc. and North-Holland Publishing Company for permission to partly reproduce our papers published in *Mathematical Bioscience* 53 : 59-77, 1981 and *Medinfo'* 80 : 427-431, 1980.

REFERENCES

1. Wagner, J.G.: *Fundamentals of clinical pharmacokinetics,* Drug Intelligence Publication, Hamilton, Illinois, 1975.
2. Buell, J., Jelliffe, R., Kalaba, R.et al.: Modern control theory and optimal drug regimens I. *Math. Biosci.* 5: 285-296, 1969.
3. Bellman, R.: Topics in pharmacolinetics III. *Math. Biosci.* 12: 1-5, 1971.
4. Koch-Weser, J.: Serum drug concentration as therapeutic guides, *New England J. Med.* 287: 227-231, 1972.
5. Kusuoka, H., Kodama, S., Maeda, H. et al.: Optimal control in compartmental systems and its application to drug administration. *Math. Biosci.* 53: 59-77, 1981.
6. Kusuoka, H., Kodama, S., Hori, M. et al.: Optimal drug administration based on a control theory, in *MEDINFO'80,* pp. 427-431, North-Holland Publ. Comp., Amsterdam, 1980.

16

ESTIMATION OF TRANSITION PROBABILITIES IN ISCHEMIC HEART DISEASE BY MARKOV MODEL

Mitsuyasu Kagiyama, Noritake Hoki, Go Tomonaga, Hideo Kusuoka, Yasuo Ogasawara and Fumihiko Kajiya

1. INTRODUCTION

In the treatment of chronic disease, its stage and severity are important, because the transition from one stage to another provides important information on the progression or regression of the disease. To evaluate transitions, changes associated with the stages must be monitored repeatedly at regular time intervals for different patient groups. This type of monitoring, however, is not always easy, especially when it requires an invasive procedure and/or the method presents technical problems. An example is monitoring the vascular lesions of ischemic heart disease (IHD), which is frequently classified as single, double, or triple vessel disease by selective coronary angiography. However, the invasiveness of coronary angiography prevents its repeated use at regular time intervals.

In the present study, we proposed a method for estimating the transition probabilities of the various stages of disease by a compartmental model. The model was applied to an analysis of the prognosis of IHD.

In clinical care, the units of the compartmental model represent various stages of the disease and the amount of tracer in a compartment represents the number of patients at a given stage. Transitions of tracers among compartments occur stochastically. In this sense, the compartmental model for evaluating the prognosis of chronic disease can be considered a common framework for the Markovian process. Several reports have indicated that the natural history of chronic disease could be modeled by the Markovian process in most cases[1-4]. In the studies reported, long-term prognosis was estimated by transition probabilities, which, as stated earlier, are not always easy to obtain.

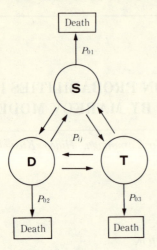

Fig. 1. Reversible 3-compartment model with an absorbing point (death). Compartments correspond to "disease states" and the amount of tracer to "the number of patients" in each state. This kind of compartmental model can be considered a common framework in the Markovian process.

In contrast to previous applications of the Markovian model, this chapter presents a method for estimating transition probabilities among stages of the disease from survival data (mortality data). According to the terms used in the Markovian model, "disease states" rather than "stages of disease" are classified as single, double, or triple vessel diseases and death. Three different types of models (one-way, catenary, and reversible) were used for the analysis (Fig. 2) and the transition probabilities among the states were estimated by the maximum likelihood method. The accuracy of identifications was evaluated by asymptotic variances and an information criterion (AIC)[7,8].

2. FORMULATION OF PROBLEM

Suppose that patients with a chronic disease are initially classified into several patient groups——disease state——by the first diagnostic procedure and that the survival data for each patient group were obtained every year for many years. Classification of the disease state cannot be performed repeatedly. The problem is to estimate transition probabilities P_{ij} among disease states from survival data. Here P_{ij} ($i \neq 0$) indicates the

(a) One Way Model (O Model)

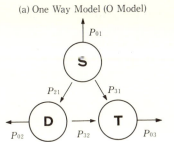

(b) Catenary Model (C Model)

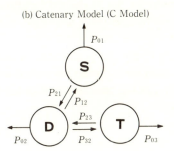

(c) Reversible Model (R Model)

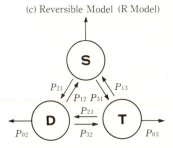

Fig. 2. Three different compartmental (Markovian) models used in the present study. The compartments (states) S, D and T denote single-, double- and triple-vessel disease, respectively. Paths to the outside of the system imply death.

transition probability from state j to state i for 1 year and P_{0j} is the probability of death from state j. The matrix P_{ij} is assumed to be time-invariant.

Consider that there are initially $N_i(0)$ patients in state i, $i=1,\cdots,n$, and that $N_i(j)$, $j=1,\cdots,t$, is the number of patients living after j years, who initially belonged in state i. In other words, $N_i(k)-N_i(k+1)$, $k=1,\cdots$,

$t-1$, represents the number of deaths during the year $k \sim k+1$, and $N_i(t)$ the number of patients alive in the tth year.

Our problem is estimating transition probabilities P_{ij} among disease states by observing $N_i(j)$, $i=1,\cdots, n$, $j=0,\cdots, t$.

3. LIKELIHOOD FUNCTION FOR SURVIVAL DATA

In this section, we derive the expression for the likelihood function to estimate P_{ij} when survival data are given by the form described in the previous section.

First, we derive the recursion formula to get the probability of death $Q_i(s)$ of a patient who initially had been in state i, during the period from $(s-1)$th year to sth year. Since $Q_i(1)$ implies the probability of death for the first one year, it is simply written as

$$Q_i(1)=P_{0i}, \quad i=1, 2, \cdots, n. \tag{1}$$

Since $Q_i(2)$ is the probability of death by way of any one of the states 1, 2, $\cdots$, and n from the initial state i, we obtain

$$Q_i(2)=\sum_{k=1}^{n} Q_k(1)P_{ki}.$$

In the same way, the recursion formula is given by

$$Q_i(s)=\sum_{k=1}^{n} Q_k(s-1)P_{ki}. \tag{2}$$

The probability that the patient will live for t years is written as

$$\bar{Q}_i(t)=1-\sum_{s=1}^{n} Q_i(s). \tag{3}$$

Using Eqs. 1-3 and considering the independent nature of the Markovian process, the likelihood of obtaining survival data $N_i(0), N_i(1),\cdots, N_i(t)$, when patients initially belonged to state i are observed is expressed by

$$L_i = \binom{N_i(0)}{N_i(0)-N_i(1)}\binom{N_i(1)}{N_i(1)-N_i(2)}\cdots\binom{N_i(t-1)}{N_i(t-1)-N_i(t)}$$
$$\times Q_i(1)^{N_i(0)-N_i(1)}Q_i(2)^{N_i(1)-N_i(2)}\cdots Q_i(t)^{N_i(t-1)-N_i(t)}\bar{Q}_i(t)^{N_i(t)}. \tag{4}$$

As the joint likelihood function L is the product of $L_1, L_2,\cdots$, and L_n, L is given by

$$L = L_1 \cdot L_2 \cdots L_n. \qquad (5)$$

4. ESTIMATING PARAMETERS

Now our problem is to estimate P_{ij} so as to maximize L in Eq. 5. However, P_{ij} has constraints based on the statistical nature of probabilities, i.e.,

$$\sum_{k=1}^{n} P_{ki} = 1 \quad \text{and} \quad 0 \leq P_{ij} \leq 1, \, i=0, 1, \cdots, n, \, j=1, \cdots, n. \qquad (6)$$

To remove the constraints in Eq. 6, parameters were transformed from P_{ij} to α_{ij}. It follows that

$$P_{ij} = \alpha_{ij}^2 \Big/ \sum_{k=0}^{n} \alpha_{kj}^2, \, i=0, 1, \cdots, n, \quad j=1, 2, \cdots, n, \qquad (7)$$

where

$$\alpha_{jj} = 1, \, j=1, 2, \cdots, n.$$

Then estimates of parameter P_{ij} are obtained by solving an ordinary non-linear optimization problem[6]. For this problem, we adopted the simplex method of Nelder and Mead[5], because it can create its own scaling factors and converge for a wide range of starting points.

5. EVALUATING THE ACCURACY OF ESTIMATES

In estimating parameters, the accuracy of the estimates must be evaluated objectively. To do this, we used the asymptotic variance obtained in the following manner.

Consider a generalized Fisher's information matrix $I(I_{kl})_{p \times p}$, where

$$I_{kl} = -E\left(\frac{\partial^2}{\partial \theta_k \partial \theta_l} \ln L\right) \qquad (8)$$

and L is the likelihood function given in Eq. 5. As a generalization of the Crámer-Rao inequality, it can be shown that the following hold: for any unbiased estimator $(\tilde{\theta}_1, \cdots, \tilde{\theta}_p)$ of $(\theta_1, \cdots, \theta_p)$, equivalent to $(P_{01}, P_{11}, \cdots)$ in our case, let V be the variance-covariance matrix. V must be larger than or equal to the matrix I^{-1} in that $V - I^{-1}$ is non-negative definite. For large samples the diagonal of I^{-1} provides an estimator for variances of maximum likelihood estimators of parameters.

Substituting Eq. 4 in Eq. 5 and taking the logarithm, it follows:

$$\log L = \sum_{k=1}^{n}\left[\sum_{s=1}^{t}(N_k(s-1)-N_k(s))\log Q_k(s) + N_k(t)\log \bar{Q}_k(t)\right]$$
$$+ (\text{the term independent of } \theta\text{'s}).\qquad(9)$$

Partially differentiating Eq. 9 with respect to θ_j, we obtain

$$\frac{\partial \log L}{\partial \theta_j} = \sum_{k=1}^{n}\left[\sum_{s=1}^{t}\frac{(N_k(s-1)-N_k(s))}{Q_k(s)}\frac{\partial Q_k(s)}{\partial \theta_j} - \frac{N_k(t)}{\bar{Q}_k(t)}\sum_{s=1}^{t}\frac{\partial Q_k(s)}{\partial \theta_j}\right]. \qquad(10)$$

Partial differentiation of Eq. 10 with respect to θ_j given

$$\frac{\partial^2 \log L}{\partial \theta_i \partial \theta_j} = \sum_{k=1}^{n}\left[\sum_{s=1}^{t}(N_k(s-1)-N_k(s))\left\{\frac{1}{Q_k(s)}\frac{\partial^2 Q_k(s)}{\partial \theta_i \partial \theta_j}\right.\right.$$
$$\left.-\frac{1}{Q_k(s)^2}\frac{\partial Q_k(s)}{\partial \theta_i}\frac{\partial Q_k(s)}{\partial \theta_j}\right\} - N_k(t)\left[\frac{1}{\bar{Q}_k(t)}\sum_{s=1}^{t}\frac{\partial^2 Q_k(s)}{\partial \theta_i \partial \theta_j}\right.$$
$$\left.\left.+\frac{1}{\bar{Q}_k(t)^2}\sum_{s=1}^{t}\frac{\partial Q_k(s)}{\partial \theta_i}\sum_{s=1}^{t}\frac{\partial Q_k(s)}{\partial \theta_j}\right\}\right]. \qquad(11)$$

Taking the expected value of Eq. 4 and making use of the following relations:

$$\langle N_k(s-1)\rangle - \langle N_k(s)\rangle = N_k(0)Q_k(s), \quad s=1,2,\cdots,t-1,$$
$$\langle N_k(t)\rangle = N_k(0)\bar{Q}_k(t). \qquad(12)$$

We have:

$$I_{ij} = \sum_{k=1}^{n}N_k(0)\left\{\sum_{s=1}^{t}\frac{1}{Q_k(s)}\frac{\partial^2 Q_k(s)}{\partial \theta_i \partial \theta_j} + \frac{1}{\bar{Q}_k(t)}\sum_{s=1}^{t}\frac{\partial Q_k(s)}{\partial \theta_i}\sum_{s=1}^{t}\frac{\partial Q_k(s)}{\partial \theta_j}\right\}. \qquad(13)$$

Since $\theta_1, \theta_2,\cdots$ correspond to transition probabilities in our problem, the partial derivatives $\partial Q_i(s)/\partial \theta_j,\cdots$ can be calculated by the following recursion formulae, which are obtained by partially differentiating Eqs. 1 and 2 with respect to θ_j:

$$\frac{\partial Q_i(1)}{\partial P_{0i}} = 1, \quad \frac{\partial Q_i(1)}{\partial P_{hk}} = 0, \quad (h,k)\neq(0,i),$$
$$\frac{\partial Q_i(t)}{\partial \theta_j} = \sum_{k=1}^{n}\frac{\partial P_{ik}}{\partial \theta_j}Q_k(s-1) + \sum_{k=1}^{n}P_{ik}\frac{\partial Q_k(s-1)}{\partial \theta_j}, \qquad(14)$$
$$t=2,3,\cdots,s, \quad i,k=1,2,\cdots n.$$

6. COMPARISON OF MODELS

In this chapter we proposed three types of models for fitting the survival data by the Markovian process. For a measure of fitness of a model, we considered applying an information criterion (AIC)[7,8], introduced by Akaike, which has been successfully applied to the identification of a statistical model.

Let $N_1, N_2, \cdots, N_t$ be the number of t independent observations of a random variable with probability density function $f(N/\Theta)$. AIC is defined as

$$\mathrm{AIC}(\Theta) = -2\sum_{i=1}^{t} \ln f(N_i/\hat{\Theta}) + 2k$$
$$= -2\ln(\text{maximum likelihood}) + 2k. \tag{15}$$

Where k is the number of independently adjustable parameters within the model and $\hat{\Theta}$ is the vector of the maximum likelihood estimates of Θ.

The model corresponding to the minimum AIC is selected as the optimal one.

7. SURVIVAL DATA FOR ISCHEMIC HEART DISEASE

Analysis of data for patients with a chronic disease is very important when estimating the natural course of the disease or comparing the effects of several treatments. This is true for ischemic heart disease (IHD) as well, and many follow-up studies of IHD have been done.

In 1973 Bruschke et al.[9] published a report on consecutive nonsurgical cases of IHD followed for 5-9 years. In their study, 553 patients were classified initially into three categories based on selective coronary angiography: single-vessel disease (S), double-vessel disease (D), and triple-vessel disease (T). The patients in each group, who survived were followed for 5-9 years.

In this study, we used Bruschke et al.'s data to estimate P_{ij} in the Markovian model, since the number of patients followed was larger than that reported by others, and their data are appropriate for an analysis of the natural history of IHD.

8. RESULTS

8.1 ESTIMATING TRANSITION PROBABILITIES
(1) Reversible model

The annual transition probabilities among S, D, T and death, calculated in the reversible model, are shown in Figure 4. Annual transition probabilities from S, D, or T states to death were 0.026, 0.090, and 0.220, respectively. These values indicated that mortality from ischemic heart disease rises steeply as the number of affected arteries increases. This model suggested that transitions from D to S or T occur with relatively high probabilities, 0.48 and 0.43, respectively, while the transition from S to D or to T occurs with low probabilities.

Results of curve fitting for survival data by the reversible model (Fig. 3) show that the three curves of mean survival values estimated for the patient groups belonged initially to states S, D, and T, respectively. These curves agreed well with the data reported by Bruschke et al.[9] For example, these authors reported 5-year survival rates of 84.8%, 61.9%, and 44.2% for the initial disease states S, D and T, respectively, while estimated values

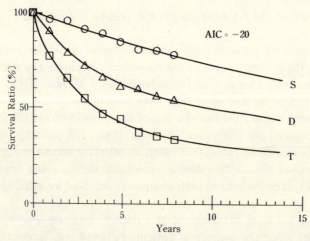

Fig. 3. Comparison of Bruschke et al.'s survival data with those estimated by applying the reversible model. The solid curves represent estimation results and the symbols ○, △ and □ are data reported by Bruschke et al. The letters S, D and T denote patient groups: single-, double-and triple-vessel diseases, respectively.

Estimation of Transition Probabilities in Ischemic Heart Disease

were 86.4%, 63.2%, and 42.5%, respectively.

(2) Catenary model

The transition probabilities obtained in the catenary model are shown in Figure 5. Although the path between S and T is neglected in the catenary model, the transition probabilities were almost compatible with those in the reversible model. The accuracy of the survival curve fit was also satisfactory.

(3) One-way model

The one-way model does not include the reversible recovery-paths of transitions, i.e., T → D, T → S and D → S. Transition probabilities calculated for this model are shown in Figure 6. The transition probabilities among S, D and T showed lower values compared with those in other models, while probabilities from S, D and T to death were almost the same as those in other models. The fit of each curve for survival data was less satisfactory.

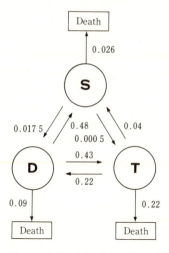

Fig. 4. Estimated values of transition probabilities in the reversible model.

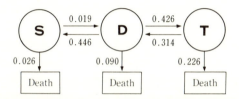

Fig. 5. Estimated values of transition probabilities in the catenary model.

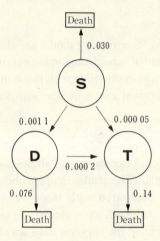

Fig. 6. Estimated values of transition probabilities in the one-way model.

8.2 COMPARISON OF THREE MODELS

The accuracy of the transition probabilities obtained for each model was evaluated by asymptotic variance, the results of which are given in the Table. 1. In general, asymptotic variance in the catenary model gave the smallest value, compared with variances for other models. The values of AIC relative to those of the one-way models are shown in the same table. The catenary model has the smallest value, indicating that this model is the most appropriate for simulating survival data.

9. DISCUSSION AND CONCLUDING REMARKS

Using three compartmental models, we analyzed the progression and regression of ischemic heart disease (IHD) in terms of single, double, and triple vessel disease and death. The estimated survival data agreed well the data reported by Bruschke et al., except for the one-way model. This suggested that IHD survival data could be modeled by a Markovian process.

After comparing the reversible model with the catenary, we selected the latter as optimal, because the AIC value and asymptotic variances were lower. That estimated transition probabilities for $S \rightleftarrows T$ also had low

Table 1. Estimated values of transition probabilities with the square roots of asymptotic variances in three different compartmental (Markovian) models. The values of AIC are given at the bottom of the Table. Note that values for both AIC and asymptotic variance are smallest for each parameter in the catenary model.

	O Model	C Model	R Model
p_{01}	0.031 ± 0.011	0.026 ± 0.009	0.026 ± 0.011
p_{21}	0.001 ± 0.65	0.019 ± 0.04	0.018 ± 0.31
p_{31}	0.000048 ± 0.32	—	0.0005 ± 0.18
p_{02}	0.0763 ± 0.013	0.902 ± 0.019	0.0904 ± 0.019
p_{12}	—	0.446 ± 0.23	0.480 ± 0.28
p_{32}	0.0002 ± 0.052	0.426 ± 0.25	0.428 ± 0.29
p_{03}	0.144 ± 0.015	0.226 ± 0.033	0.225 ± 0.039
p_{13}	—	—	0.0419 ± 0.30
p_{23}	—	0.314 ± 0.13	0.220 ± 0.68
AIC	0	-24	-20

values, supports this selection.

On transition probabilities in the catenary model, values for paths from T to D were relatively high, indicating that coronary artery lesions may regress in the chronic course of IHD. However, the regression does not necessarily imply only morphological improvement in the vascular lesion; it also includes functional improvement. Progression of the disease from D to T will be rapid because its transition probability was higher than that from S to D.

The present study indicates that the Markovian model provides useful information for evaluating prognosis in chronic disease, based on survival data.

REFERENCES

1   Inoue, M., Kajiya, F, Hori, M. et al.: Clinical Pharmacology and System Theory. Proc. 14th Int. Sym. on Clinical Pharmacology, 316-334, 1977.
2   Hori, M. Kitabatake, A., Inoue, M. et al.: Prediction of long-term prognosis of chronic diseases based on the Markov chain. ICCS-78 Tokyo. 54-59, 1978.
3   Kagiyama, M., Hoki, N., Tomonaga, G. et al.: Estimation of the state transition probabilities in coronary heart disease by Markov model. World Congress on Med. Phys. & Bio. Eng. Hamburg. 584, 1982.
4   Urakabe, S., Orita, Y., Shirai, D. et al.: Prognosis of chronic glomerulonephritis in adult patients estimated on the basis of the Markov process. *Clin. Nephrol.* 3: 130-149, 1975.
5   Nelder, J.A. & Mead, R.: A simplex method for function minimization. *Comput. J.* 7: 308-

313, 1965.
6 Jacoby, S.L.S., Kowalik, J.S. & Pizzo, J.T.: Iterative methods for nonlinear optimization problems. New Jersey, Prentice-Hall Inc. 1972.
7 Akaike, H.: A new look at the statistical model identification, *IEEE Trans.* AC-19: 716-723, 1974.
8 Akaike, H.: Information theory and an extension of the maximum likelihood principle. 2nd Int. Symp. Inform. Theory, 267-281, 1973.
9 Bruschke, A.V.G., Proudfit, W.L. & Sones, F.M.: Progress study of 590 consecutive non-surgical cases of coronary disease followed 5-9 years. 1. Arteriographic correlations. *Circulation* 47: 1147-1153, 1973

Index

Accuracy of estimates 30
Active transport 136
  secondary 136
AIC (an information criterion) 10, 12, 181, 184
Anger camera 91
Argon gas 97
Arteriovenous oxygen difference (A−V)O_2 102
Asymptotic variance 15, 19, 23, 26, 33, 34, 179, 184
^{198}Au colloids 142

Blood circulatory system 59
Brownian motion 159

Calcium 139
Canonical form 48
Cardiac output 59, 61, 63
Catenary model 177
Catenary system 33, 48, 52
Cerebral
  blood flow (CBF) 97, 101
  circulation 97
  metabolic rate of oxygen (CMRO$_2$) 102
  oxygen consumption 97
  vascular resistance (CVR) 102
Chronic pulmonary emphysema 131
Circulatory system 62
Closed system 37
Compartmental matrix 3
Compartmental system, time-discrete model 3
Complex complicance 126, 130

Compliance 126
Concentration of drug
  mean 168, 170, 172
  minimal effective 168, 170, 171
  peak 168, 171, 172
Constancy of tracer mass 10
Continuous distribution 127, 129
  model 119
Controllability 5
Coronary
  angiography 175, 181
  stenosis 72
Creatine kinase (CK) 79
^{51}Cr RBC 142
  survival 149
Cramer-Rao inequality 23, 179
Cyclical system 17, 33

dead space 131
  ventilation 132
Disease state 176
Distribution function 119, 121, 125, 126, 128, 130
Distribution of
  compliance 132
  lung volume 121, 124, 130, 131
  mechanical time constant 131
  pulmonary blood flow 121
  pulmonary ventilation 124
  ventilation 121, 130
  washout time constant 122
Divalent cation 106, 114, 116
Driving point (DP) system 39, 40, 42, 43
Drug dosage

maintenance 170, 171, 172
  total 170, 171, 172
Dual system 43

Electrolyte metabolism 135
Enzyme 79
Estimation of
  infarct size 83
  parameter 9
Exponential function 10
Extracellular fluid 138

Fallout 156, 162
Fick's
  equation 127
  principle 67, 99
Fisher's information 23, 32, 179
Flow rate of tracer 2
Food chain 156
Fourier transform method 10
Functional image 90

Health physics 156
Height over area method 71
Henry's law 99
Hereditary spherocyte 144
Homeomorphism 38, 39
Hydrogen gas clearance method 66

Identifiability 5
  necessary and sufficient condition for the structural 43
  necessary conditions for structural 40
  parameter 36
  structural 36, 38
Identification 5
  of parameter 17
  problem 10
^{131}I hippuran 90
^{131}I labeled human serum albumin (RIHSA) 59
Impulse response 167
Indicator dilution method 59
Inert gas 127, 129

Initial slope method 71
Input-output data 10
Interstitial fluid 138
Intracardiac shunt flow 60
Intracellular fluid 138
Intrasplenic compartments
  fast path 145
  intermediate pool 145
  slow pool 145
Inulin space 138
Iron 139
Ischemic heart disease (IHD) 175
Ito calculus 156, 159

Kety's equation 67

Labyrinthine block 139
Least squares estimation 10
Likelihood function 12, 17, 24, 32, 178
Linear compartmental system 3, 9, 31
Lung volume 121

Magnesium 139
Mammillary system 48, 52
Markov parameters 39
Markovian process 175
Mass transport process 59
Matrix 32
Maximum likelihood 11, 23
Mean arterial blood pressure (MAP) 101
Mean blood flow rate 61
Mean transit time 62
Mechanical time constant 125, 126, 132
Microsphere 66, 69
Miniature end-plate potential (min. e. p. p.) 106-114, 116
Minimal realization 54
Moments method 10
Multiple regression analysis, spleen hemodynamic parameters 151
Myocardial
  CK, function of appearance 81
  CK-MB isoenzyme 81
  infarction 80

Neuromuscular preparation 106
Nitrogen washout test, lung 122
Non-oscillatory 167
   compartmental system 166
Nonlinear optimization 18, 179
Number of compartment 5, 9
N_2 washout 125, 130

Observability 5
One way model 177, 183
Open system 37
Optimal
   control 5
   drug administration 166
   sampling condition 5, 23
   sampling interval 27, 30, 34
Oxygen delivery (O_2DEL) 102

Parameter estimation 62
Partition coefficient 128
   blood-gas 68
   brain-blood 99
Passive diffusion 136
Peeling method 10
Pharmacokinetic study 4
Plasma volume 138
^{210}Po metabolism 156, 162
Poisson
   distribution 10, 23, 32
   fluctuation 19
Post-tetancic rise 109
Post-tetanic increase 106
Potassium 139
Precursor compartment 92, 93
Prony's method 10
Pulmonary
   blood flow 121
   function 119, 133
   gas exchange 121

Radioactive renogram 90
Radiocardiogram (RCG) 59
Radiocardiorgraphy 59
Radionuclide 156
Radiosplenogram

   by intra-arterial injection 145
   by intra-venous injection 145
Rate constant 5, 9
Reachability 5
Realizability 5, 49
   of driving point functions 50
   of transfer functions 51
Receiving compartment 40
Recirculation 146
Red blood cell 136
Red cell deformability 153
Regional myocardial blood flow 66
Renal hemodynamics 90
Renogram
   C_{max} 91, 93
   Down slope 91, 93
   T_{max} 91, 93
   Up slope 91, 93
Respiratory quotient (RQ) 102
Retention ratio 128, 129, 130
Reversible model 177, 182
Rhodan space 138
RI (radioisotope) 10, 23, 59
   count 17
   data 32
   tracer kinetic data 11

Sampling condition
   smaple size 26
   sampling interval 3, 26
Serum CK determination 83
Serum enzyme 79
Shunt flow rate 61
Simplex method 12, 18, 179
Sink 40
Sodium 135, 139
Sodium space 138
Source 40
Spleen circulation
   cell elements 142
   plasma 142
Spleen perfusion 142
Splenic blood flow
   by Xe-133 washout 149
   by heat-denatured red cells clear-

Index

ance 149
Stochastic input 156, 158, 162
  stationary 161
Stroke care unit 98
Sufficiently connectedness 39
  necessary conditions for 41
Survival data 176

^{99m}Tc HSA 142
Temperature 107-109, 111-116
Tetanic stimulation 106, 107, 109, 111, 113, 114
Transfer (T)
  system 39-42, 45
  coefficient 156, 158
Transit 40
Transition probability 176, 182
Tree-compartmental
  analysis 145

system 52

Urodynamics 90

Vascular lesion 175
Ventilation 121, 133
Ventilation-to-perfusion ratio 127, 133
Volume-elastic unit 126

Washout time constant 124, 125, 130, 131
Water
  heavy 137
  total body 137
  metabolism 135
White noise 157, 161

^{133}Xe clearance technique 66